Do You Ever Wish You Could . . .

. . . Lose weight rapidly?

. . . Drop a dress size or two within a matter of weeks?

. . . Stay motivated on a diet and not get bored?

. . . Be more energetic and not so tired all the time?

. . . Feel better about yourself and your appearance almost right away?

. . . Not look and feel so bloated?

. . . Exercise less and still lose weight?

. . . Have people come up to you and ask you what diet you're on to look that great?

. . . See important health numbers like LDL cholesterol, blood pressure, and blood sugar start to drop?

. . . Stay at your goal weight with no more yo-yoing up and down?

. . . Enjoy yourself on weekends and not have to watch every morsel you put in your mouth?

If you answered yes to any of these questions,
The 17 Day Diet and *The 17 Day Diet Workbook* are for you!

The 17 Day Diet Workbook

Your Guide to Healthy Weight Loss
with Rapid Results

DR. MIKE MORENO

FREE PRESS

New York   London   Toronto   Sydney   New Delhi

Disclaimer: This publication is intended to provide helpful and informative material. It is not intended to diagnose, treat, cure, or prevent any health problem or condition, nor is intended to replace the advice of a physician. No action should be taken solely on the contents of this book. Always consult your physician or qualified health-care professional on any matters regarding your health and before adopting any suggestions in this book or drawing inferences from it.

The author and publisher specifically disclaim all responsibility for any liability, loss, or risk, personal or otherwise, which is incurred as a consequence, directly or indirectly, from the use or application of any contents of this book.

Any and all product names referenced within this book are the trademarks of their respective owners. None of these owners have sponsored, authorized, endorsed, or approved this book. Always read all information provided by the manufacturers' product labels before using their products. The author and publisher are not responsible for claims made by manufacturers. The statements made in this book have not been evaluated by the Food and Drug Administration.

*f*P

FREE PRESS
A Division of Simon & Schuster, Inc.
1230 Avenue of the Americas
New York, NY 10020

Copyright © 2011 by 17 Day Diet, Inc.

First Free Press hardcover edition August 2011

FREE PRESS and colophon are trademarks of Simon & Schuster, Inc.

For information about special discounts for bulk purchases, please contact Simon & Schuster Special Sales at 1-866-506-1949 or business@simonandschuster.com.

The Simon & Schuster Speakers Bureau can bring authors to your live event. For more information or to book an event contact the Simon & Schuster Speakers Bureau at 1-866-248-3049 or visit our website at www.simonspeakers.com.

Manufactured in the United States of America

1   3   5   7   9   10   8   6   4   2

ISBN 978-1-4516-6143-9

Contents

· · · · · · · · · · · ·

Get Started

• • • • • • • • • • • • •

Welcome to *The 17 Day Diet Workbook*—a practical, easy-to-use guide that supports *The 17 Day Diet*. The 17 Day Diet is a four-cycle program designed to take weight off *rapidly*. Isn't that what we all want? Absolutely—hardly anyone I know, or any of my patients, likes to *endure* depressingly slow weight loss. We want to be trim now . . . look great now . . . and feel great now. That's what the 17 Day Diet does—it gets you to where you want to be quickly, without a lot of sacrifice, hunger pangs, or cravings. The diet is nutritionally sound, too, it's easy to follow, and it works. I call it the best thing since the sliced bread you'll give up (but for only the first two cycles).

How Fast Can I Lose Weight?

I've seen people lose up to 10 to 12 pounds the first 17 days, and keep losing steadily right down to their goals. The beauty of this program is that you won't get discouraged or bored by the prospect of staying on a diet for what seems like forever—because you'll be shedding fat so quickly. You'll love the fact that in seven, 10, or 17 days, you'll be slimmer. And if your results are like so many others, you'll feel a lot lighter and have an absurd amount of energy.

The 17 Day Diet really is simple and effective. Of course, you'll keep a few "forbidden foods" off your plate for the first three cycles, but feel free to enjoy all the rest.

What Is Forbidden?

Forbidden isn't really the right word, because nothing is off limits after the first three cycles. But the foods you will ban temporarily—and later reintroduce only sparingly—are foods like bread, pasta, and anything made with flour.

You'll also want to become a stranger to sugary sodas, fruit juices and drinks, jams, jellies, baked goods, and many desserts.

How Is the Diet Structured?

The beauty of the 17 Day Diet is that it works in four cycles, depending on how much weight you'd like to lose.

Cycle 1 is the initial 17-day period in which you give up all bread, rice, potatoes, pasta, baked goods, fruit, candy, cake, ice cream, and alcohol. It's the strictest period, but also when the most rapid weight loss occurs. And it's easier than you think. You won't even miss carbs after a few days—your body gets used to not relying on them. You get to eat unlimited amounts of certain proteins and vegetables. And you'll supplement your daily diet with probiotics like yogurt and kefir—foods shown in research to help the body burn fat.

The great thing about Cycle 1 is that you can use it anytime: when you need to break a plateau, get back to your goal weight, fit into a smaller dress size for the weekend or a swimsuit for a cruise—any time you want to accelerate your weight loss and do it safely. Cycle 1 is one of your best quick-weight-loss resources.

During Cycle 2, you slowly begin to reintroduce certain carbs back into the diet, such as legumes, whole grains, and starchy vegetables, along with lots of other foods. Weight loss continues, and still fairly rapidly. And now you can drink a little wine—something most diets forbid.

On Cycle 3, you get to eat a huge array of healthy foods: breads, more meats, more starches, and fun foods like low-carb frozen dessert treats. You ease off some of the strictness of the first two cycles while still continuing to knock off pounds. Every 17 days you're changing things up so that you never get bored. Every day is exciting, because you see the results on your scale or in your looser-fitting clothes.

Cycle 4 is the maintenance period that, ideally, you stay on the rest of your life. It lets you stay at your new weight as long as you do two things: enjoy yourself on the weekend, and use your favorite cycle during the week. So once you're happy with your new svelte self, continue to enjoy occasional forbidden foods. Just do so carefully or you'll find yourself back on a slippery slope to your prediet Pudge Town. If you fall off the wagon for a weekend or, say, on a vacation, don't panic. Just jump back to Cycle 1 to quickly shave any weight you gain.

You Mean I Can Cheat?

Yes, on the weekends, if you want to! If you stay on your favorite cycle during the week—that's when it's easiest to "diet"—you can stray off track a bit on the weekends. Come Monday morning, you simply minimize any damage by getting back on one of the cycles.

Why Does the 17 Day Diet Work So Well?

Scientifically, eliminating unhealthy foods from your system keeps them from making a beeline to your belly and elsewhere. Healthy foods do the opposite. The higher amounts of lean protein you eat, for example, boost your metabolism in a number of physiologically active ways. This diet is high in fiber, too. Fiber is an appetite suppressant, a detoxifier, and a food component that ushers bad calories out of your system before they have time to camp out on your thighs. Then there is the addition of probiotics, now believed to keep fat formation in check.

Another reason the 17 Day Diet works is because you're changing your calorie count and the foods you eat. By varying these things, you keep your body and metabolism guessing. I call this "body confusion." The scale is less likely to get stuck. The added bonus: You'll never get bored. And it's fun watching those pounds melt off. So confusion is good!

But, more important, the 17 Day Diet works because it's realistic. Nothing derails a diet faster than distressing round-the-clock hunger pangs, or boredom. But the 17 Day Diet isn't about depriving yourself of food or variety. I encourage you to eat until you are no longer hungry—and even snack between meals—as long as you're eating the right foods. That doesn't mean just broccoli, either. Nuts, cheeses, and other delicious foods are permitted as you progress through the cycles. There are so many choices, too, that you'll never get bored on this plan.

Okay, Let's Cut to the Chase!

You've read this and you're a believer, yet you can't wait to get started. To learn all the intricacies of how and why the diet works, you really need to get the book, *The 17 Day Diet*. But if you can't get to the bookstore right away, here's an overview:

Quick and Easy Overview of the 17 Day Diet	
Cycles	**Purpose**
Cycle 1: Accelerate (17 days)	To promote rapid weight loss by improving digestive health. It helps clear sugar from the blood to boost fat-burning and discourage fat storage.
Cycle 2: Activate (17 days)	To reset your metabolism through a strategy that involves increasing and decreasing your caloric consumption to stimulate fat-burning and to help prevent plateaus.
Cycle 3: Achieve (17 days)	To develop good eating habits through the reintroduction of additional foods and move you closer to your goal weight.
Cycle 4: Arrive (ongoing)	To keep you at your goal weight through a program of eating that lets you enjoy your favorite foods on weekends, while eating healthfully during the week.

Using This Workbook

. . . .

For losing weight on the 17 Day Diet, this journal is indispensable. You'll use it to keep track of your eating, exercise, strategies, goals, and milestones—all motivational information. Once you start writing things down, you'll see patterns that start to emerge, you'll overcome obstacles to weight loss, and you'll feel empowered to make positive changes to your life and your health.

I've made all of this simple for you with pages on which you can record information quickly and easily. Part of the format includes simple checklists designed to save time.

Once you get the hang of journaling, you'll love it—and the motivation it gives you to be your best ever.

Here's a summary of the practical tools you'll find in *The 17 Day Diet Workbook*:

Get Motivated

Start the workbook and the 17 Day Diet by recording your motivations to lose weight. The more motivated you feel, the more success you'll have. Revisit this section often, especially if you need a nudge to keep going.

Your Starting Point and Goal Weight

You'll enter your starting weight and post pictures of yourself here. Then I'll help you find a realistic goal for your body type.

Daily Meal Planner

Yes, you must write down everything you eat, even if it's not on the diet. Then you can look back and say, "Wow, I ate six cream-filled donuts on Tuesday. No wonder I'm not losing weight."

I want you to be brutally honest, and accountable to yourself. If you're going to fudge the truth about fudge, why even bother to keep a journal packed with fibs?

Here are some examples of *honest* entries:

> *Entry 1: Breakfast: yogurt and an apple. Note: I wanted to reach for a big chocolate chip cookie, but that would be like having whiskey at 9 a.m. Deviant behavior successfully avoided.*
>
> *Entry 2: Horrible day! At midnight I ate a box of cookies with two bowls of ice cream. Let's go for total failure.*

Seriously, you're less likely to have entries like that last one if you make journaling a regular practice. You'll think twice about eating something bad if you have to put it down on paper. Writing down what you eat each day practically guarantees weight-loss success. In fact, dieters who record daily what they eat drop twice as much weight as those who don't, according to research. No one will read your workbook but you—so at least try journaling for the first 17 days and see if your eating habits improve.

Daily Exercise Planner

While following the 17 Day Diet, plan on moving your body more (trips to the fridge don't count). I've included an exercise log on which you will record strength-training and cardio workouts. Please use this to:

- Plan out your workouts (in other words, write out each workout at least a day in advance). Planning always leads to personal accountability.

- Fill in the spaces that ask you for progress benchmarks such as duration, calories burned, poundages lifted, and so forth.

- Analyze your workouts at least once a week. Note where you've improved: you're lifting heavier weights, jogging farther, or pushing yourself to work out longer than 17 minutes. Seeing your progress on paper is incredibly motivating.

Reflection

Along the way, I'll ask you a series of probing questions. Don't worry; they're for your eyes only, and there will not be a test. Write down what's working and what's not working. What did you do well? Where do you need to improve? These sections will help you stay on track and change nonproductive habits.

Review

After each cycle, you'll assess your success and prepare for your transition to the next cycle of the 17 Day Diet. I'll also ask you to consider any strategies for change.

Also in *The 17 Day Diet Workbook*:

Recipes

I've got 17 brand-new, mouthwatering recipes for you to help guide your menu decisions. They take less than 30 minutes to whip together, and are geared for the four cycles of this program.

Shopping List

This features an expanded list of foods and shows you how to shop for weight-loss success. Each food is matched to its appropriate cycle.

Food Guide

We don't count calories or nutrients on the 17 Day Diet per se, but this mini food guide gives you important nutritional information on the foods you'll be eating.

Exercise Guide

Since exercise burns calories, this section shows you how many calories are burned per hour in any number of activities, from attending an aerobic dance class to pulling weeds in your garden. Consult this chart to see how many calories you're burning through exercise, then record that number in your exercise planner.

Tips

Every day I'll give a tip to help you stay on track. To use this journal successfully, you can start with a few basic tips now:

1. Correctly follow the 17 Day Diet instructions.
2. Purchase *The 17 Day Diet* book.
3. Take before, during, and after photos.
4. Use and fill in this journal daily.

Along the way, I'll show you how to critically analyze what your journal reveals. This is so important, since most of us live on the surface, never touching any depth. Many people are just too busy to listen to the world inside them and spend too much time listening to the world outside them. To journal takes silence, reflection, and slowing down.

Now for a few specifics to get you started on the right track. . . .

Get Motivated

••••••••••••••••••

I'm sure you have many reasons why you want to lose weight, but the most important one is you and your quality of life. In the space below, write down all the reasons (including that one!) and motivations for losing weight—and keeping it off. Revisit your writings here at least once a week, or whenever you feel your motivation waning.

My Motivation

_____

_____

_____

_____

Why Losing Weight Matters to Me

_____

_____

_____

_____

_____

_____

My Motivation

Why Losing Weight Matters to Me

My Motivation

Why Losing Weight Matters to Me

My Motivation

Why Losing Weight Matters to Me

My Motivation

Why Losing Weight Matters to Me

My Motivation

Why Losing Weight Matters to Me

My Motivation

Why Losing Weight Matters to Me

Your Starting Point and Goal Weight

Y ou can't get anywhere if you don't know where you're going. I'm sure your goal is to drop approximately a whole lot of weight, preferably in the form of fat, but water will do as long as it brings results on the scale. The key is to set a realistic and attainable weight for your frame. With an appropriate goal ahead of you, you're much more likely to continue—and even look forward to—your plan. Goal setting improves the possibility of success and boosts positive psychological changes in self-confidence and motivation.

How Much Should You Weigh?

As you begin the 17 Day Diet, select a specific weight goal—a weight at which you feel you will look your best. Keep in mind that there's really no such thing as the "perfect" weight because we all come in a variety of body shapes, heights, and bone structures. There are, however, ideal weight ranges, so there is a simple equation I tend to follow:

If you're a woman: Take 100 pounds for the first five feet of your height, and add five pounds for each extra inch to get the midpoint of what your ideal body weight range should be. Then you need to factor in your body structure. Some people are smaller boned; others are big boned. If you're small boned, I subtract 15 percent from the normal-frame weights; if you're large boned, I add 15 percent to the normal-frame weights. For a lot of people, that's too much math. So I did the math for you:

WOMEN		
Small-Boned Frame	**Midpoint**	**Large-Boned Frame**
5' = 85	**5' = 100**	5' = 115
5' 1" = 90	**5' 1" = 105**	5' 1" = 121
5' 2" = 94	**5' 2" = 110**	5' 2" = 127
5' 3" = 98	**5' 3" = 115**	5' 3" = 132
5' 4" = 102	**5' 4" = 120**	5' 4" = 137
5' 5" = 106	**5' 5" = 125**	5' 5" = 144
5' 6" = 110	**5' 6" = 130**	5' 6" = 150
5' 7" = 115	**5' 7" = 135**	5' 7" = 155
5' 8" = 119	**5' 8" = 140**	5' 8" = 161
5' 9" = 123	**5' 9" = 145**	5' 9" = 167
5' 10" = 128	**5' 10" = 150**	5' 10" = 173
5' 11" = 132	**5' 11" = 155**	5' 11" = 178
6' = 136	**6' = 160**	6' = 184

If you're a man: Take 110 pounds for the first five feet of your height and add six pounds for each extra inch to get the midpoint of what should be your ideal body weight range. The men's chart appears on the opposite page. Allow for being small or large boned, as explained above.

A caveat: These charts are only rough estimates with a large range of variability. We are all made differently, and there is not one ideal weight for every height. Base your goal on a weight at which you feel and look your best—a goal also approved by your doctor.

Write It Down!

I've always been a goal setter. I love the idea of writing down what I want to achieve and then watching my life improve as I make the changes necessary to make that goal a reality. I've never accomplished

MEN		
Small-Boned Frame	*Midpoint*	*Large-Boned Frame*
5' = 94	5' = 110	5' = 127
5' 1" = 99	5' 1" = 116	5' 1" = 133
5' 2" = 104	5' 2" = 122	5' 2" = 140
5' 3" = 109	5' 3" = 128	5' 3" = 147
5' 4" = 114	5' 4" = 134	5' 4" = 154
5' 5" = 119	5' 5" = 140	5' 5" = 161
5' 6" = 124	5' 6" = 146	5' 6" = 168
5' 7" = 129	5' 7" = 152	5' 7" = 175
5' 8" = 134	5' 8" = 158	5' 8" = 182
5' 9" = 139	5' 9" = 164	5' 9" = 189
5' 10" = 145	5' 10" = 170	5' 10" = 196
5' 11" = 150	5' 11" = 176	5' 11" = 202
6' = 155	6' = 182	6' = 209
6' 1" = 160	6' 1" = 188	6' 1" = 216
6' 2" = 165	6' 2" = 194	6' 2" = 223
6' 3" = 170	6' 3" = 200	6' 3" = 230
6' 4" = 175	6' 4" = 206	6' 4" = 237
6' 5" = 180	6' 5" = 212	6' 5" = 244
6' 6" = 185	6' 6" = 218	6' 6" = 251

a goal without significant benefits to my life in ways I didn't antici-pate. (There is, however, a downside to being a goal setter. When the project is complete, the goal achieved, I feel a little adrift. I end up having a significant discussion with myself about what's next and why.) Anyway, in the space below, please write down your goal weight (and expect to achieve it!).

My Starting Weight	Be sure to weigh yourself on the morning you start the 17 Day Diet. Record your weight in the box at the left.
My Goal Weight	Using the charts above, select a goal weight. Enter it in the box at the left. I'll ask you to monitor your progress toward your goal all the way through the 17 Day Diet.

Let Me Ask You . . .

About your weight goals, I'd like you to consider some of the issues below before you get started. Then write out your answers.

1. **Your desired weight:**

   Why do you want to be at this weight?

   _____

   _____

   _____

   _____

   _____

   What is special about this weight?

   _____

   _____

   _____

   _____

   _____

2. **Past weight goals:**

   Have you set weight goals in the past?

   _____

   _____

   _____

   _____

   _____

Were they different from this goal? If yes, why?

_____

_____

_____

_____

_____

3. **Your weight history:**

When were you last at your desired weight?

_____

_____

_____

_____

_____

What could keep you from staying at that weight?

_____

_____

_____

_____

_____

How would you avoid those obstacles?

_____

_____

_____

_____

_____

4. **Getting to your goal:**

How important is it to get to your goal?

_____

_____

_____

_____

_____

If it is important, why?

_____

_____

_____

_____

_____

5. **Not getting to your goal:**

How would you feel if you didn't reach your desired goal?

_____

_____

_____

_____

_____

What effect would it have on your self-confidence, health and fitness, social life, personal relationships, and other aspects of daily life?

_____

_____

_____

_____

_____

Really think about your answers. What you write can often hold solutions to achieving what you desire in life. Come back to this part of the journal if you ever find yourself slipping.

Visual Motivation: Take Before and After Photos

Take a picture of yourself before you start the 17 Day Diet. Follow up by taking pictures after every cycle in the same outfit, whether a bathing suit or workout clothing, and then compare. You may not realize the changes your body is making on a daily basis, but the photographs can put things into perspective. Finally, take an "After" photo when you reach your goal.

Paste your photos in the spaces below.

Before

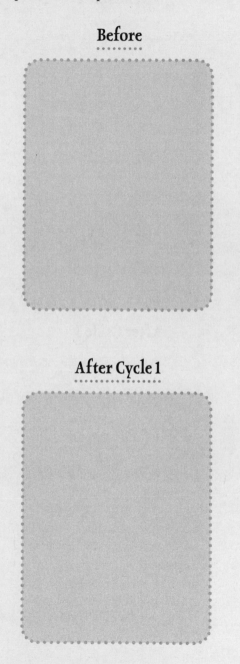

After Cycle 1

After Cycle 2

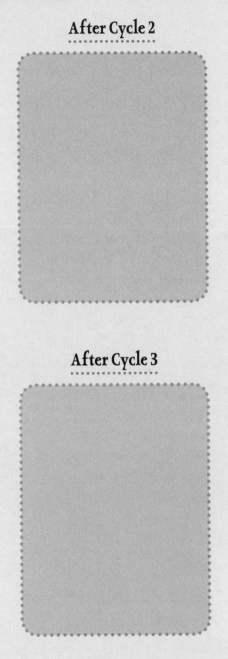

After Cycle 3

After Cycle 4 or at Your Goal Weight

Incentives

Whenever possible, create incentives to help you reach your goals. For example, if you want to lose weight, buy an expensive outfit that's several sizes too small. The thought of having a beautiful outfit unused in your closet can be an effective impetus to keep you going. Or hang it up on your door so you can see it every day. On a weekly basis, try it on and see how it fits. If you can barely fit into it, wait and then try it on again later. Alternatively, suggest to your spouse or partner that you be taken on a romantic vacation if you reach your self-determined goal. Getting others involved in your weight-loss effort builds a support network that can spur you on to greater heights.

Visualize Your Success

Visualization is a technique that can be used to reinforce goals and sustain your motivation. Essentially, it is an organized form of daydreaming. Many athletes use this technique to actualize their potential. A basketball player, for instance, might visualize swishing a last-second jump shot, or a baseball player might visualize hitting a game-winning home run. The technique works beautifully in fitness and weight loss, where it has been demonstrated to increase motivation and adherence to a program.

This approach is best practiced in a quiet environment without any distractions. Close your eyes and relax your muscles. Begin to think about your physique. Visualize each problem area—abs, butt, thighs, and so forth—and get an image of the way you want them to look. Picture yourself in great shape, walking on the beach in a bikini or wearing a sexy dress at an event. Make the image as clear and realistic as possible, seeing it as a movie in your head.

You might even want to think of a person whose physique you admire, such as a famous celebrity, fitness model, or perhaps even someone who works out in your gym. Fantasize that you possess the body of your role model and carry this vision with you. Let your imagination be your internal source of motivation.

This journal is designed to make losing weight on the 17 Day Diet more personal, more fun, more motivating, and ultimately, more successful. What you learn about yourself over the four cycles of this program can carry over into a lifetime of good health and a healthy weight. You've got all it takes. It's all right here, and within you. Now . . . here's an amazing four-cycle plan to help you get lean, fit, strong, and motivated.

CYCLE 1

· · · · · · · · · · · · · · · · · ·

Accelerate

GOAL

To trigger rapid weight loss in a healthy manner by mobilizing fat stores and flushing water and toxins from your system.

What to Eat: The Accelerate Cycle Food List

Lean Proteins

Here's where you'll be getting a lot of your fat-burning power. Eat all you want of the following proteins. They're freebies. The 17 Day Diet is purposely high in protein because protein stimulates the reduction of body fat.

Fish*

Canned light tuna *(in water)*

Catfish

Flounder

Haddock

Halibut

Herring

Perch *(ocean)*

Salmon, canned or fresh

Sardines *(canned in mustard or tomato sauce, not oil)*

Shad

Sole

Tilapia

Trout *(freshwater)*

Tuna

---

*See the Food Guide on pages 301–314 for other fish allowed in Cycle 1. Opt for wild-caught rather than farm-raised fish, which may have received doses of antibiotics. Avoid shark, swordfish, king mackerel, tilefish, grouper, marlin, and orange roughy. They are the most likely to carry metals like methylmercury, which is considered a toxin.

Poultry

Chicken breasts

Turkey breasts

Ground turkey, lean

Eggs *(2 eggs = 1 serving)*

Egg whites *(4 egg whites = 1 serving)*

Cleansing Vegetables

Eat all you want from the following list. They're freebies, too. I call these "cleansing vegetables" because they support detoxification in the intestines, blood, and liver, and offer protective antioxidants.

Artichoke

Artichoke hearts

Asparagus

Bell peppers: green, orange, red, yellow

Broccoli

Brussels sprouts

Cabbage

Carrots

Cauliflower

Celery

Cucumbers

Eggplant

Garlic

Green beans

Green, leafy vegetables *(including beet greens, turnip greens, collard greens)*

Kale

Leeks

Lettuce, all varieties

Mushrooms

Okra

Onions

Parsley

Scallions

Spinach
Tomatoes
Watercress

Low-Sugar Fruit—2 servings daily

Low-sugar fruits are good sources of fiber, which provides bulk and digests slowly, helping you feel full. They're also full of water and super low in calories, which makes them ideal for weight loss.

Apples
Berries, all types
Grapefruit
Oranges
Peaches
Pears
Plums
Prickly pear cactus
Prunes
Red grapes

Probiotic Foods—2 servings daily

Probiotics help balance your digestive system, resulting in an overall increase in the efficiency of digestion. Research shows that probiotics may also help fight obesity. There's no recommended daily allowance for probiotics. To maintain health, 5–10 billion is adequate. That may sound like a lot, but consider this: a 6-ounce serving of yogurt contains around 17 billion probiotics.

Yogurt, any type, including Greek-style, sugar-free fruit flavored, plain, and low-fat *(6-ounce container = 1 serving)*
Kefir: similar to a drinking-style yogurt; great for making smoothies *(1 cup = 1 serving)*
Low-fat acidophilus milk *(1 cup = 1 serving)*
Yakult: *(1 small 50-calorie bottle = 1 serving)*

Breakstone's LivActive cottage cheese *(½ cup = 1 serving)*

Reduced salt miso dissolved in low-fat, low-sodium broth

(1 tablespoon = 1 serving)

Tempeh (a fermented cake of pressed soybeans) *(4 ounces = 1 serving)*

Sauerkraut *(½ cup = 1 serving)*

Kimchi *(Korean cabbage) (½ cup = 1 serving) Find it in Asian supermarkets or natural food stores, and enjoy a small amount as a side dish with meals.*

Friendly Fats—1 to 2 tablespoons daily

Olive oil

Flaxseed oil

Condiments

Condiments and seasonings are allowed in moderation: salsa, low-carb marinara sauce, lite soy sauce, reduced-sugar ketchup, fat-free sour cream, low-fat, low-sodium broth, Truvia (a noncaloric sweetener made from natural ingredients), sugar-free jams and jellies, vegetable cooking spray, fat-free cheeses (i.e., Parmesan), fat-free salad dressing, salt, pepper, vinegar, mustard, herbs, and spices.

Meal Planning Made Easy

It's easy to remember what to eat during this cycle:

- Have as much as you want of specific proteins and cleansing vegetables.
- Supplement these foods with 2 low-sugar fruits daily; 2 servings of probiotic foods such as yogurt, kefir, Yakult, acidophilus milk, reduced-salt miso dissolved in low-fat, low-sodium broth, and sauerkraut (½ cup a serving); and 1 to 2 tablespoons of friendly fats. It's that easy.

You do not have to count anything, except your 2 daily fruit servings, your 2 daily probiotic servings, and your fat serving.

Here is a sample menu on the Accelerate Cycle.

Wake-up drink

Every morning, as soon as you rise, drink one 8-ounce cup of hot water. Squeeze half a lemon into the cup; the lemon stimulates your digestive juices. Your goal is to drink at least seven more glasses of water by the end of the day.

Day 1

Breakfast
- 2 scrambled egg whites
- ½ grapefruit, or other fresh fruit
- 1 cup green tea

Lunch
- Large green salad topped with tuna; drizzle with 1 tablespoon olive or flaxseed oil and 2 tablespoons balsamic vinegar
- 1 cup green tea

Dinner
- Plenty of grilled chicken with liberal amounts of any vegetables from the list, steamed or raw
- 1 cup green tea

Snacks
- 6 ounces of sugar-free plain yogurt mixed with 1–2 tablespoons sugar-free jam; or other probiotic serving
- 1 serving of fruit from the list

DAY 1—MY DAILY FOOD CHART   DATE

Dr. Mike's Food Tip of the Day

Start thinking like a weight-loss winner. To be successful, you have to overcome the self-defeating thoughts that plague people trying to lose weight. Don't set unrealistic goals you can't control. Be positive about what you can do. If you slip, ignore it and continue with your program. Find the hidden triggers that cause you problems, and avoid these triggers.

WEIGHT

WATER INTAKE

number of 8-ounce glasses

☐ ☐ ☐ ☐
☐ ☐ ☐ ☐

FOOD INTAKE

number of servings

☐ Lean Proteins

☐ Cleansing Vegetables

☐ Low-Sugar Fruit (2 servings)

☐ Probiotic Foods (2 servings)

☐ Friendly Fats (1–2 tablespoons)

Breakfast

_____
_____
_____
_____
_____

Lunch

_____
_____
_____
_____

Dinner

_____
_____
_____
_____

Snacks

_____
_____
_____

Dr. Mike's Workout Tip of the Day

Exercising at lower levels of exertion encourages the body to burn fat, so go easy on yourself! It's Day 1 of Cycle 1, so all you need to do is get in 17 minutes of easy exercising today, like walking around your neighborhood or inside a nearby mall.

Cardio

DATE	ACTIVITY DESCRIPTION	DURATION	CALORIES BURNED	DISTANCE	STEPS

Toning Exercises

EXERCISES	SETS	REPS	WEIGHT	TIME	CALORIES BURNED

DAY 1—MY DAILY JOURNAL

What worked well?

_____
_____
_____

What didn't work well?

_____
_____
_____

I experienced the following challenges:

_____
_____
_____

**Ways to overcome these challenges
(brainstorm as many problem-solvers as you can):**

_____
_____
_____

**From your list, choose the best solutions and develop
strategies for success.**

_____
_____
_____

Reflections: Journal how you're feeling, your successes, anything that comes to mind about your progress so far. Read through *The 17 Day Diet* book to learn about all my strategies for overcoming barriers. Which ones can you apply today?

_____
_____
_____
_____
_____
_____
_____

DAY 2—MY DAILY FOOD CHART   DATE

Dr. Mike's Food Tip of the Day

Leaner, stronger, healthier—that's what eating vegetables will do for your body! Dieters who eat the widest variety of veggies have the least amount of body fat, according to a Tufts University study. So get thin, not flabby. Eat as many of the cleansing vegetables as you want during Cycle 1 of the 17 Day Diet.

WEIGHT

WATER INTAKE

number of 8-ounce glasses

☐ ☐ ☐ ☐
☐ ☐ ☐ ☐

FOOD INTAKE

number of servings

☐ Lean Proteins

☐ Cleansing
   Vegetables

☐ Low-Sugar Fruit
   (2 servings)

☐ Probiotic Foods
   (2 servings)

☐ Friendly Fats
   (1–2 tablespoons)

Breakfast

Lunch

Dinner

Snacks

Dr. Mike's Workout Tip of the Day

As you complete your 17-minute workout today, visualize the new you—the "you" with the trained, toned physique who is active, healthy, and enjoying life. Keep this picture in your mind as you make it happen, day by day.

Cardio

DATE	ACTIVITY DESCRIPTION	DURATION	CALORIES BURNED	DISTANCE	STEPS

Toning Exercises

EXERCISES	SETS	REPS	WEIGHT	TIME	CALORIES BURNED

DAY 2—MY DAILY JOURNAL

What worked well?

_____

_____

_____

What didn't work well?

_____

_____

_____

I experienced the following challenges:

_____

_____

_____

Ways to overcome these challenges
(brainstorm as many problem-solvers as you can):

_____

_____

_____

From your list, choose the best solutions and develop
strategies for success.

_____

_____

_____

Reflections: Journal how you're feeling, your successes, anything that
comes to mind about your progress so far. Read through *The 17 Day Diet*
book to learn about all my strategies for overcoming barriers. Which
ones can you apply today?

_____

_____

_____

_____

_____

_____

DAY 3—MY DAILY FOOD CHART   DATE

Dr. Mike's Food Tip of the Day

Fruit is good for you, right? Yes, it is, but certain fruits like pineapple, watermelon, and bananas are high in sugar and do not promote fat loss. So choose low-sugar fruits—berries, apples, oranges, and grapefruit—throughout Cycle 1. Only two servings a day, please, and consume them before 2 p.m. Fruit is a carb and timing of carbohydrate intake is important!

WEIGHT

WATER INTAKE

number of 8-ounce glasses

☐ ☐ ☐ ☐
☐ ☐ ☐ ☐

FOOD INTAKE

number of servings

☐ Lean Proteins

☐ Cleansing Vegetables

☐ Low-Sugar Fruit (2 servings)

☐ Probiotic Foods (2 servings)

☐ Friendly Fats (1–2 tablespoons)

Breakfast

_____
_____
_____
_____

Lunch

_____
_____
_____

Dinner

_____
_____
_____
_____

Snacks

_____
_____
_____

Dr. Mike's Workout Tip of the Day

Think of your 17-minute workout not as "work" but as 17 minutes of moving your body and doing something you enjoy. Are you a fan of one of the dance shows on TV, like *Dancing with the Stars* or *So You Think You Can Dance*? Do *you* like to dance? Put on your favorite music and move!

Cardio

DATE	ACTIVITY DESCRIPTION	DURATION	CALORIES BURNED	DISTANCE	STEPS

Toning Exercises

EXERCISES	SETS	REPS	WEIGHT	TIME	CALORIES BURNED

DAY 3—MY DAILY JOURNAL

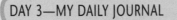

What worked well?

_____

_____

_____

_____

What didn't work well?

_____

_____

_____

_____

I experienced the following challenges:

_____

_____

_____

**Ways to overcome these challenges
(brainstorm as many problem-solvers as you can):**

_____

_____

_____

**From your list, choose the best solutions and develop
strategies for success.**

_____

_____

_____

Reflections: Journal how you're feeling, your successes, anything that
comes to mind about your progress so far. Read through *The 17 Day Diet*
book to learn about all my strategies for overcoming barriers. Which
ones can you apply today?

_____

_____

_____

_____

_____

_____

DAY 4—MY DAILY FOOD CHART   DATE

Dr. Mike's Food Tip of the Day

As I explained in *The 17 Day Diet* book, bugs can be good for you! Good "bugs" or bacteria help your digestive tract form a barrier against bad bacteria. That's why I suggest two servings a day of the friendly type of bacteria called probiotics. Found in yogurt, kefir, miso, tempeh, and others, these good guys also help you lose weight!

WEIGHT

WATER INTAKE

number of 8-ounce glasses

☐ ☐ ☐ ☐
☐ ☐ ☐ ☐

FOOD INTAKE

number of servings

☐ Lean Proteins

☐ Cleansing Vegetables

☐ Low-Sugar Fruit (2 servings)

☐ Probiotic Foods (2 servings)

☐ Friendly Fats (1–2 tablespoons)

Breakfast

_____
_____
_____
_____
_____

Lunch

_____
_____
_____
_____

Dinner

_____
_____
_____
_____
_____

Snacks

_____
_____
_____

Dr. Mike's Workout Tip of the Day

If you're working out on your own, put your gym times on your daily calendar. And think about getting your workouts in early. I have found that people who get up in the morning and exercise the first thing tend to stay with programs longer. They get it over with and feel so much better the rest of the day.

Cardio

DATE	ACTIVITY DESCRIPTION	DURATION	CALORIES BURNED	DISTANCE	STEPS

Toning Exercises

EXERCISES	SETS	REPS	WEIGHT	TIME	CALORIES BURNED

DAY 4—MY DAILY JOURNAL

What worked well?

_____

_____

_____

What didn't work well?

_____

_____

_____

I experienced the following challenges:

_____

_____

_____

**Ways to overcome these challenges
(brainstorm as many problem-solvers as you can):**

_____

_____

_____

**From your list, choose the best solutions and develop
strategies for success.**

_____

_____

_____

Reflections: Journal how you're feeling, your successes, anything that
comes to mind about your progress so far. Read through *The 17 Day Diet*
book to learn about all my strategies for overcoming barriers. Which
ones can you apply today?

_____

_____

_____

_____

_____

_____

DAY 5—MY DAILY FOOD CHART   DATE

Dr. Mike's Food Tip of the Day

How many times have you been told that you should drink eight 8-ounce glasses of water each day? A thousand times? Well, now you've been told a thousand and one times! And here's why: Drinking water is essential to weight loss and helps your body metabolize stored fat. It also helps the body flush waste from your system and is the best solution for fluid retention.

WEIGHT

WATER INTAKE

number of 8-ounce glasses

☐ ☐ ☐ ☐
☐ ☐ ☐ ☐

FOOD INTAKE

number of servings

☐ Lean Proteins

☐ Cleansing
   Vegetables

☐ Low-Sugar Fruit
   (2 servings)

☐ Probiotic Foods
   (2 servings)

☐ Friendly Fats
   (1–2 tablespoons)

Breakfast

_____
_____
_____
_____

Lunch

_____
_____
_____
_____

Dinner

_____
_____
_____
_____

Snacks

_____
_____
_____

Dr. Mike's Workout Tip of the Day

Have you recruited a workout buddy? The accountability your spouse, your children, or a friend from work can provide can keep you going when you'd rather just collapse in the recliner. So, buddy up with someone for your 17-minute workout whenever possible. It's a lot harder to talk yourself out of exercising when someone else is counting on you!

Cardio

DATE	ACTIVITY DESCRIPTION	DURATION	CALORIES BURNED	DISTANCE	STEPS

Toning Exercises

EXERCISES	SETS	REPS	WEIGHT	TIME	CALORIES BURNED

DAY 5—MY DAILY JOURNAL

What worked well?

_____
_____
_____

What didn't work well?

_____
_____
_____

I experienced the following challenges:

_____
_____
_____

**Ways to overcome these challenges
(brainstorm as many problem-solvers as you can):**

_____
_____
_____

**From your list, choose the best solutions and develop
strategies for success.**

_____
_____
_____

Reflections: Journal how you're feeling, your successes, anything that
comes to mind about your progress so far. Read through *The 17 Day Diet*
book to learn about all my strategies for overcoming barriers. Which
ones can you apply today?

_____
_____
_____
_____
_____
_____
_____

DAY 6—MY DAILY FOOD CHART   DATE

Dr. Mike's Food Tip of the Day

Whoops! Do I see you recording the iced tea you had with lunch toward your daily water intake? Sorry, but coffee and tea do not count toward your eight glasses of water . . . neither do diet sodas, regular sodas, energy drinks, juice, sports drinks, or flavored waters, but feel free to add a lemon or lime wedge to good ol' H_2O.

WEIGHT

WATER INTAKE

number of 8-ounce glasses

☐ ☐ ☐ ☐
☐ ☐ ☐ ☐

FOOD INTAKE

number of servings

☐ Lean Proteins

☐ Cleansing
Vegetables

☐ Low-Sugar Fruit
(2 servings)

☐ Probiotic Foods
(2 servings)

☐ Friendly Fats
(1–2 tablespoons)

Breakfast

_____
_____
_____
_____
_____

Lunch

_____
_____
_____
_____
_____

Dinner

_____
_____
_____
_____

Snacks

_____
_____
_____

Dr. Mike's Workout Tip of the Day

Break it up! If 17 minutes at one time seems challenging at first, try breaking up your workout into two manageable parts. Maybe you can fit in a 10-minute walk over your lunch hour, then take a short (at least 7-minute) bike ride after dinner. Whatever it takes, get your body used to moving for a minimum of 17 minutes every day, without fail.

Cardio

DATE	ACTIVITY DESCRIPTION	DURATION	CALORIES BURNED	DISTANCE	STEPS

Toning Exercises

EXERCISES	SETS	REPS	WEIGHT	TIME	CALORIES BURNED

DAY 6—MY DAILY JOURNAL

What worked well?

_____
_____
_____

What didn't work well?

_____
_____
_____

I experienced the following challenges:

_____
_____
_____

Ways to overcome these challenges
(brainstorm as many problem-solvers as you can):

_____
_____
_____

From your list, choose the best solutions and develop
strategies for success.

_____
_____
_____

Reflections: Journal how you're feeling, your successes, anything that comes to mind about your progress so far. Read through *The 17 Day Diet* book to learn about all my strategies for overcoming barriers. Which ones can you apply today?

_____
_____
_____
_____
_____
_____

DAY 7—MY DAILY FOOD CHART   DATE

Dr. Mike's Food Tip of the Day

What's so special about green tea? Besides water, green tea is a beverage of choice, thanks to certain chemicals it contains that increase fat-
burning and stimulate the calorie-burning process. New research
suggests that something in green tea inhibits a process of blood vessel
growth that can cause fat tissue to grow. In light of all this, drinking
three cups of green tea daily is highly recommended.

WEIGHT

WATER INTAKE

number of 8-ounce glasses

☐ ☐ ☐ ☐
☐ ☐ ☐ ☐

FOOD INTAKE

number of servings

☐ Lean Proteins

☐ Cleansing
Vegetables

☐ Low-Sugar Fruit
(2 servings)

☐ Probiotic Foods
(2 servings)

☐ Friendly Fats
(1–2 tablespoons)

Breakfast

Lunch

Dinner

Snacks

Dr. Mike's Workout Tip of the Day

Stretch your muscles for a minute or two after exercises. This helps ease your body into your workout by slowly increasing your heart rate and breathing. Cooling down is also important since stopping abruptly can cause dizziness, cramping, or muscle soreness.

Cardio

DATE	ACTIVITY DESCRIPTION	DURATION	CALORIES BURNED	DISTANCE	STEPS

Toning Exercises

EXERCISES	SETS	REPS	WEIGHT	TIME	CALORIES BURNED

DAY 7—MY DAILY JOURNAL

What worked well?

_____
_____
_____

What didn't work well?

_____
_____
_____

I experienced the following challenges:

_____
_____
_____

**Ways to overcome these challenges
(brainstorm as many problem-solvers as you can):**

_____
_____
_____

**From your list, choose the best solutions and develop
strategies for success.**

_____
_____
_____

Reflections: Journal how you're feeling, your successes, anything that
comes to mind about your progress so far. Read through *The 17 Day Diet*
book to learn about all my strategies for overcoming barriers. Which
ones can you apply today?

_____
_____
_____
_____
_____
_____
_____

DAY 8—MY DAILY FOOD CHART   DATE

Dr. Mike's Food Tip of the Day

Fats can actually help you burn fat! Not all fats are bad guys, like the trans fats found in processed foods and the saturated fats found in animal products. Friendly fats are the polyunsaturated ones mostly found in fish and vegetable oils. Omega-3 fatty acids, for example, boost your metabolism. In Cycle 1, choose salmon or canned light tuna (in water). For cooking, choose olive or flaxseed oil (1–2 table-spoons daily).

WEIGHT

WATER INTAKE

number of 8-ounce glasses

☐ ☐ ☐ ☐
☐ ☐ ☐ ☐

FOOD INTAKE
number of servings

☐ Lean Proteins

☐ Cleansing
  Vegetables

☐ Low-Sugar Fruit
  (2 servings)

☐ Probiotic Foods
  (2 servings)

☐ Friendly Fats
  (1–2 tablespoons)

Breakfast

_____
_____
_____
_____
_____

Lunch

_____
_____
_____
_____

Dinner

_____
_____
_____
_____

Snacks

_____
_____
_____

Dr. Mike's Workout Tip of the Day

Stay safe while walking outdoors by wearing brightly colored clothes and facing any approaching traffic. Riding a bike? The same defensive measures apply, plus a few more. Avoid potential injuries by wearing a helmet and making sure you can be seen by vehicles. Use a light and attach reflectors on your bike's wheels for added safety.

Cardio

DATE	ACTIVITY DESCRIPTION	DURATION	CALORIES BURNED	DISTANCE	STEPS

Toning Exercises

EXERCISES	SETS	REPS	WEIGHT	TIME	CALORIES BURNED

DAY 8—MY DAILY JOURNAL

What worked well?

_____

_____

_____

What didn't work well?

_____

_____

_____

I experienced the following challenges:

_____

_____

_____

**Ways to overcome these challenges
(brainstorm as many problem-solvers as you can):**

_____

_____

_____

**From your list, choose the best solutions and develop
strategies for success.**

_____

_____

_____

Reflections: Journal how you're feeling, your successes, anything that
comes to mind about your progress so far. Read through *The 17 Day Diet*
book to learn about all my strategies for overcoming barriers. Which
ones can you apply today?

_____

_____

_____

_____

_____

_____

DAY 9—MY DAILY FOOD CHART   DATE

Dr. Mike's Food Tip of the Day

Fresh or dried herbs and spices can add flavor and pizzazz to your meals. Basil and oregano can add an Italian flavor, while a sprinkling of cumin and chili powder add a Mexican flair. Try a dash of curry for an Indian taste, or combine ginger with lite soy sauce for an Asian taste-bud treat. Experiment! There is no reason for your meals to be bland and tasteless!

WEIGHT

WATER INTAKE

number of 8-ounce glasses

☐ ☐ ☐ ☐
☐ ☐ ☐ ☐

FOOD INTAKE

number of servings

☐ Lean Proteins

☐ Cleansing Vegetables

☐ Low-Sugar Fruit (2 servings)

☐ Probiotic Foods (2 servings)

☐ Friendly Fats (1–2 tablespoons)

Breakfast

_____
_____
_____
_____
_____

Lunch

_____
_____
_____
_____

Dinner

_____
_____
_____
_____

Snacks

_____
_____
_____

Dr. Mike's Workout Tip of the Day

Variety is the spice of life, and that also applies to your workout. Even if you really enjoy walking, change it up a couple days a week to keep things interesting. Try dusting off that badminton set in the garage and playing a few games after dinner with the kids. Sign up for a ballroom dance class or a water aerobics session.

Cardio

DATE	ACTIVITY DESCRIPTION	DURATION	CALORIES BURNED	DISTANCE	STEPS

Toning Exercises

EXERCISES	SETS	REPS	WEIGHT	TIME	CALORIES BURNED

DAY 9—MY DAILY JOURNAL

What worked well?

_____
_____
_____

What didn't work well?

_____
_____
_____

I experienced the following challenges:

_____
_____
_____

**Ways to overcome these challenges
(brainstorm as many problem-solvers as you can):**

_____
_____
_____

**From your list, choose the best solutions and develop
strategies for success.**

_____
_____
_____

Reflections: Journal how you're feeling, your successes, anything that
comes to mind about your progress so far. Read through *The 17 Day Diet*
book to learn about all my strategies for overcoming barriers. Which
ones can you apply today?

_____
_____
_____
_____
_____
_____

DAY 10—MY DAILY FOOD CHART   DATE

Dr. Mike's Food Tip of the Day

The more planning you do, the better off you will be. Before you leave the house, grab a snack to take with you, like a piece of fruit, so you're not running through the drive-through instead. Stock up on healthy foods. No, Diet Coke and reduced-fat Twinkies don't count. Try new things, like raw spinach, a new fruit, or not stuffing yourself silly at buffets. Keep healthy snacks around you. Then hire bouncers to keep you away from all the spots where you hid all the unhealthy treats.

WEIGHT

WATER INTAKE

number of 8-ounce glasses

☐ ☐ ☐ ☐
☐ ☐ ☐ ☐

FOOD INTAKE

number of servings

☐ Lean Proteins

☐ Cleansing
   Vegetables

☐ Low-Sugar Fruit
   (2 servings)

☐ Probiotic Foods
   (2 servings)

☐ Friendly Fats
   (1–2 tablespoons)

Breakfast

_____
_____
_____
_____
_____

Lunch

_____
_____
_____
_____

Dinner

_____
_____
_____
_____

Snacks

_____
_____
_____

Dr. Mike's Workout Tip of the Day

Do you think of yourself as a good listener? If so, make sure you are listening to your body, too! That means paying attention to sudden, sharp pains or prolonged fatigue. There is a difference between that "good tired" feeling that follows a brisk walk and the kind of tired that lets you know you've overdone it.

Cardio

DATE	ACTIVITY DESCRIPTION	DURATION	CALORIES BURNED	DISTANCE	STEPS

Toning Exercises

EXERCISES	SETS	REPS	WEIGHT	TIME	CALORIES BURNED

DAY 10—MY DAILY JOURNAL

What worked well?

_____
_____
_____

What didn't work well?

_____
_____
_____

I experienced the following challenges:

_____
_____
_____

Ways to overcome these challenges
(brainstorm as many problem-solvers as you can):

_____
_____
_____

From your list, choose the best solutions and develop
strategies for success.

_____
_____
_____

Reflections: Journal how you're feeling, your successes, anything that
comes to mind about your progress so far. Read through *The 17 Day Diet*
book to learn about all my strategies for overcoming barriers. Which
ones can you apply today?

_____
_____
_____
_____
_____
_____

DAY 11—MY DAILY FOOD CHART   DATE

Dr. Mike's Food Tip of the Day

Think you can't live without ketchup or sour cream? Condiments, in moderation, may be incorporated into your Cycle 1 diet. Just choose the low-carb ketchup, fat-free sour cream, and sugar-free jams and jellies. Salsa, lite soy sauce, fat-free salad dressings and cheeses, vinegar, mustard, and vegetable cooking spray can also be on your grocery list. I also give a thumbs-up to Truvia, a noncaloric sweetener made from natural ingredients.

WEIGHT

WATER INTAKE

number of 8-ounce glasses

☐ ☐ ☐ ☐
☐ ☐ ☐ ☐

FOOD INTAKE

number of servings

☐ Lean Proteins

☐ Cleansing
   Vegetables

☐ Low-Sugar Fruit
   (2 servings)

☐ Probiotic Foods
   (2 servings)

☐ Friendly Fats
   (1–2 tablespoons)

Breakfast

_____

_____

_____

_____

_____

Lunch

_____

_____

_____

_____

Dinner

_____

_____

_____

_____

Snacks

_____

_____

_____

Dr. Mike's Workout Tip of the Day

Don't get discouraged! If you have been a couch potato for months or years, you can't expect to be ready to run a marathon in a week or two. However, by recording your workouts, you'll be able to track the progress you've made and soon will begin to feel it.

Cardio

DATE	ACTIVITY DESCRIPTION	DURATION	CALORIES BURNED	DISTANCE	STEPS

Toning Exercises

EXERCISES	SETS	REPS	WEIGHT	TIME	CALORIES BURNED

DAY 11—MY DAILY JOURNAL

What worked well?

_____

_____

_____

What didn't work well?

_____

_____

_____

I experienced the following challenges:

_____

_____

_____

**Ways to overcome these challenges
(brainstorm as many problem-solvers as you can):**

_____

_____

_____

**From your list, choose the best solutions and develop
strategies for success.**

_____

_____

_____

Reflections: Journal how you're feeling, your successes, anything that comes to mind about your progress so far. Read through *The 17 Day Diet* book to learn about all my strategies for overcoming barriers. Which ones can you apply today?

_____

_____

_____

_____

_____

_____

DAY 12—MY DAILY FOOD CHART   DATE

Dr. Mike's Food Tip of the Day

If you find it difficult to get in two servings of probiotic foods each day, or just don't care for them, feel free to substitute one or both servings with a probiotic supplement. Just make sure it contains 10 to 20 billion colony-forming units (CFUs) and store it as instructed on the label.

WEIGHT

WATER INTAKE

number of 8-ounce glasses

☐ ☐ ☐ ☐
☐ ☐ ☐ ☐

FOOD INTAKE

number of servings

☐ Lean Proteins

☐ Cleansing Vegetables

☐ Low-Sugar Fruit (2 servings)

☐ Probiotic Foods (2 servings)

☐ Friendly Fats (1–2 tablespoons)

Breakfast

_____
_____
_____
_____
_____

Lunch

_____
_____
_____
_____

Dinner

_____
_____
_____
_____

Snacks

_____
_____
_____

Dr. Mike's Workout Tip of the Day

Think you are too stressed out to exercise? Once you start exercising on a daily basis, you will find yourself feeling more relaxed and less stressed. Increased activity through exercise causes the brain to release more serotonin, a natural mood elevator, and can be the best remedy when you feel depression coming on.

Cardio

DATE	ACTIVITY DESCRIPTION	DURATION	CALORIES BURNED	DISTANCE	STEPS

Toning Exercises

EXERCISES	SETS	REPS	WEIGHT	TIME	CALORIES BURNED

DAY 12—MY DAILY JOURNAL

What worked well?

_____

_____

_____

What didn't work well?

_____

_____

_____

I experienced the following challenges:

_____

_____

_____

Ways to overcome these challenges
(brainstorm as many problem-solvers as you can):

_____

_____

_____

From your list, choose the best solutions and develop
strategies for success.

_____

_____

_____

Reflections: Journal how you're feeling, your successes, anything that
comes to mind about your progress so far. Read through *The 17 Day Diet*
book to learn about all my strategies for overcoming barriers. Which
ones can you apply today?

_____

_____

_____

_____

_____

_____

_____

DAY 13—MY DAILY FOOD CHART   DATE

Dr. Mike's Food Tip of the Day

If you're taking statins—prescription drugs taken to lower cholesterol—you may think eating grapefruit is off limits. While it's true that an interaction was discovered in the nineties, the amount and the time of day it is consumed is key. Consult your doctor about whether you might eat a limited amount of grapefruit (i.e., ½ grapefruit) in the morning and then take statins in the evening.

WEIGHT

WATER INTAKE

number of 8-ounce glasses

☐ ☐ ☐ ☐
☐ ☐ ☐ ☐

FOOD INTAKE

number of servings

☐ Lean Proteins

☐ Cleansing
   Vegetables

☐ Low-Sugar Fruit
   (2 servings)

☐ Probiotic Foods
   (2 servings)

☐ Friendly Fats
   (1–2 tablespoons)

Breakfast

_____
_____
_____
_____
_____

Lunch

_____
_____
_____
_____
_____

Dinner

_____
_____
_____
_____

Snacks

_____
_____
_____

Dr. Mike's Workout Tip of the Day

Today's best reason to complete your 17-minute workout: It slows down some aspects of the aging process. While your peers may begin to experience aches and pains from inactivity, you will be strengthening your muscles and joints and improving your flexibility and your ability to maintain an active lifestyle.

Cardio

DATE	ACTIVITY DESCRIPTION	DURATION	CALORIES BURNED	DISTANCE	STEPS

Toning Exercises

EXERCISES	SETS	REPS	WEIGHT	TIME	CALORIES BURNED

DAY 13—MY DAILY JOURNAL

What worked well?

_____
_____
_____

What didn't work well?

_____
_____
_____

I experienced the following challenges:

_____
_____
_____

Ways to overcome these challenges
(brainstorm as many problem-solvers as you can):

_____
_____
_____

From your list, choose the best solutions and develop
strategies for success.

_____
_____
_____

Reflections: Journal how you're feeling, your successes, anything that
comes to mind about your progress so far. Read through *The 17 Day Diet*
book to learn about all my strategies for overcoming barriers. Which
ones can you apply today?

_____
_____
_____
_____
_____
_____

DAY 14—MY DAILY FOOD CHART   DATE

Dr. Mike's Food Tip of the Day

Even though you are free to use 1–2 tablespoons of olive or flaxseed oil daily as a "friendly fat," 1 tablespoon of any kind of oil contains 14 grams of fat. Instead, use fat-free cooking spray to drastically cut fat from your diet. There are several varieties, including olive oil and canola oil. For stir-fry dishes that require higher heat, look for a "professional" cooking spray, designed to be used at high temperatures.

WEIGHT

WATER INTAKE

number of 8-ounce glasses

☐ ☐ ☐ ☐
☐ ☐ ☐ ☐

FOOD INTAKE

number of servings

☐ Lean Proteins

☐ Cleansing Vegetables

☐ Low-Sugar Fruit (2 servings)

☐ Probiotic Foods (2 servings)

☐ Friendly Fats (1–2 tablespoons)

Breakfast

Lunch

Dinner

Snacks

Dr. Mike's Workout Tip of the Day

Are you sick and tired of being sick and tired? Exercise boosts immune function so you will come down with fewer colds and bounce back from them sooner. This boost comes from improved blood flow, which flushes away toxins from muscles and organs. It also helps remove germs and circulates antibodies that fight infection.

Cardio

DATE	ACTIVITY DESCRIPTION	DURATION	CALORIES BURNED	DISTANCE	STEPS

Toning Exercises

EXERCISES	SETS	REPS	WEIGHT	TIME	CALORIES BURNED

DAY 14—MY DAILY JOURNAL

What worked well?

_____

_____

_____

What didn't work well?

_____

_____

_____

I experienced the following challenges:

_____

_____

_____

Ways to overcome these challenges
(brainstorm as many problem-solvers as you can):

_____

_____

_____

From your list, choose the best solutions and develop
strategies for success.

_____

_____

_____

Reflections: Journal how you're feeling, your successes, anything that
comes to mind about your progress so far. Read through *The 17 Day Diet*
book to learn about all my strategies for overcoming barriers. Which
ones can you apply today?

_____

_____

_____

_____

_____

_____

_____

DAY 15—MY DAILY FOOD CHART   DATE

Dr. Mike's Food Tip of the Day

Natural list-makers start each day with a "to do" list. Are you one of them? If you aren't already doing your grocery shopping from a list, now's the time to start! Before you enter your supermarket, make sure you have your list. Include all the food items you will need for the coming week, based on the 17 Sample Menus from *The 17 Day Diet* or create your own based on guidelines in the book. Check out my comprehensive Shopping List, beginning on page 265.

WEIGHT

WATER INTAKE

number of 8-ounce glasses

☐ ☐ ☐ ☐
☐ ☐ ☐ ☐

FOOD INTAKE

number of servings

☐ Lean Proteins

☐ Cleansing
Vegetables

☐ Low-Sugar Fruit
(2 servings)

☐ Probiotic Foods
(2 servings)

☐ Friendly Fats
(1–2 tablespoons)

Breakfast

_____
_____
_____
_____
_____

Lunch

_____
_____
_____
_____

Dinner

_____
_____
_____
_____

Snacks

_____
_____

Dr. Mike's Workout Tip of the Day

Do you need to go shoe shopping? Having the right type of exercise shoes is so important and often overlooked until foot problems begin to appear. Shop for a shoe that fits well, with room for your toes to wiggle freely. Your heel should not slide in and out of the shoe when tied tightly, and should be designed for your particular activity.

Cardio

DATE	ACTIVITY DESCRIPTION	DURATION	CALORIES BURNED	DISTANCE	STEPS

Toning Exercises

EXERCISES	SETS	REPS	WEIGHT	TIME	CALORIES BURNED

DAY 15—MY DAILY JOURNAL

What worked well?

_____
_____
_____

What didn't work well?

_____
_____
_____

I experienced the following challenges:

_____
_____
_____

Ways to overcome these challenges
(brainstorm as many problem-solvers as you can):

_____
_____
_____

From your list, choose the best solutions and develop
strategies for success.

_____
_____
_____

Reflections: Journal how you're feeling, your successes, anything that
comes to mind about your progress so far. Read through *The 17 Day Diet*
book to learn about all my strategies for overcoming barriers. Which
ones can you apply today?

_____
_____
_____
_____
_____
_____

DAY 16—MY DAILY FOOD CHART   DATE

Dr. Mike's Food Tip of the Day

Removing the skin on chicken and turkey reduces fat content more than you might think. A 3.5-ounce portion of roasted chicken contains 13.6 grams of fat with skin, 7.4 grams without skin. That same portion of white meat turkey is 6.3 grams of fat with skin, 3.2 grams of fat without skin. Choosing dark meat turkey ups the fat ante to 11.5 grams of fat with, 7.2 grams without.

WEIGHT

WATER INTAKE

number of 8-ounce glasses

☐ ☐ ☐ ☐
☐ ☐ ☐ ☐

FOOD INTAKE

number of servings

☐ Lean Proteins

☐ Cleansing
   Vegetables

☐ Low-Sugar Fruit
   (2 servings)

☐ Probiotic Foods
   (2 servings)

☐ Friendly Fats
   (1–2 tablespoons)

Breakfast

_____
_____
_____
_____
_____

Lunch

_____
_____
_____
_____

Dinner

_____
_____
_____
_____
_____

Snacks

_____
_____
_____

Dr. Mike's Workout Tip of the Day

Exercise clothing for warm-weather and indoor workouts should be comfortable and lightweight. Look for clothing that breathes well, dries quickly, and allows you to move your body freely. Clothing should be insulating to keep you warm. Dress in layers with a lightweight, breathable layer closest to the skin, followed by an insulating top layer.

Cardio

DATE	ACTIVITY DESCRIPTION	DURATION	CALORIES BURNED	DISTANCE	STEPS

Toning Exercises

EXERCISES	SETS	REPS	WEIGHT	TIME	CALORIES BURNED

DAY 16—MY DAILY JOURNAL

What worked well?

_____

_____

_____

What didn't work well?

_____

_____

_____

I experienced the following challenges:

_____

_____

_____

**Ways to overcome these challenges
(brainstorm as many problem-solvers as you can):**

_____

_____

_____

**From your list, choose the best solutions and develop
strategies for success.**

_____

_____

_____

Reflections: Journal how you're feeling, your successes, anything that
comes to mind about your progress so far. Read through *The 17 Day Diet*
book to learn about all my strategies for overcoming barriers. Which
ones can you apply today?

_____

_____

_____

_____

_____

_____

DAY 17—MY DAILY FOOD CHART   DATE

Dr. Mike's Food Tip of the Day

Check the nutrition facts of foods labeled fat-free. They are not always a healthy choice! When fat is removed, sugar is sometimes added. The result is a food that is high in calories and low in nutrients.

WEIGHT

WATER INTAKE

number of 8-ounce glasses

☐ ☐ ☐ ☐
☐ ☐ ☐ ☐

FOOD INTAKE

number of servings

☐ Lean Proteins

☐ Cleansing Vegetables

☐ Low-Sugar Fruit (2 servings)

☐ Probiotic Foods (2 servings)

☐ Friendly Fats (1–2 tablespoons)

Breakfast

_____
_____
_____
_____
_____

Lunch

_____
_____
_____
_____

Dinner

_____
_____
_____
_____

Snacks

_____
_____

Dr. Mike's Workout Tip of the Day

Walking is the best form of exercise for just about everyone. It requires no equipment (except those shoes I just talked about), is a low-impact exercise and can be done indoors or outdoors. Your 17-minute daily walk can reduce your heart attack risk by the same percentage as your jogging friends.

Cardio

DATE	ACTIVITY DESCRIPTION	DURATION	CALORIES BURNED	DISTANCE	STEPS

Toning Exercises

EXERCISES	SETS	REPS	WEIGHT	TIME	CALORIES BURNED

DAY 17—MY DAILY JOURNAL

What worked well?

_____

_____

_____

What didn't work well?

_____

_____

_____

I experienced the following challenges:

_____

_____

_____

Ways to overcome these challenges
(brainstorm as many problem-solvers as you can):

_____

_____

_____

From your list, choose the best solutions and develop
strategies for success.

_____

_____

_____

Reflections: Journal how you're feeling, your successes, anything that comes to mind about your progress so far. Read through *The 17 Day Diet* book to learn about all my strategies for overcoming barriers. Which ones can you apply today?

_____

_____

_____

_____

_____

_____

Review: Weight-Loss Checklist—Cycle 1

•••

Do any of these apply to you? Read through these statements and answer (truthfully!) to gauge your progress during Cycle 1.

1. Am I accurately recording everything I am eating?

   ☐ **Always**   ☐ **Sometimes**   ☐ **Rarely or Never**

2. Am I weighing myself three to four days a week?

   ☐ **Always**   ☐ **Sometimes**   ☐ **Rarely or Never**

3. Am I eating regular meals and snacks as outlined in *The 17 Day Diet*?

   ☐ **Always**   ☐ **Sometimes**   ☐ **Rarely or Never**

4. Am I eating the proper foods on this cycle?

   ☐ **Always**   ☐ **Sometimes**   ☐ **Rarely or Never**

5. Am I completing at least 17 minutes of daily exercise?

   ☐ **Always**   ☐ **Sometimes**   ☐ **Rarely or Never**

My top areas to work on in the next cycle:

_____

_____

_____

_____

I lost _____ pounds on Cycle 1.

How do you feel about your weight loss?

_____

_____

_____

_____

CYCLE 2

· · · · · · · · · · · · · · · · · ·

Activate

What to Eat: The Activate Cycle Food List

On the Activate Cycle, you'll be adding new foods to those you ate on the Accelerate Cycle. These additional foods are listed below.

Proteins

Add in the following foods:

Shellfish

Clams
Crab
Lobster
Mussels
Oysters
Scallops
Shrimp

Lean Cuts* of Meat

The leanest cuts are those from the part of the animal that gets the most exercise. Therefore, cuts from the round, chuck, shank, and flank are the best.

Beef round tip
Beef top loin
Beef top sirloin
Eye of the round
Flank steak

---

*Lean cuts tend to be a little tougher. You can tenderize lean cuts by marinating in fat-free liquids like fruit juice, wine, fat-free salad dressings, or fat-free broth.

Ground beef, lean
Lamb shanks
Lamb sirloin roast
Pork boneless loin roast
Pork sirloin chops
Pork tenderloin
Pork top or center loin chops
Top round
Top sirloin steak
Veal cutlet

Natural Starches

Grains (1 serving = ½ cup)

Amaranth
Barley, pearled
Brown rice
Bulgur
Couscous
Cream of Wheat
Grits
Longer grain rice, such as basmati
Millet
Oat bran
Old-fashioned oatmeal
Quinoa

Legumes (1 serving = ½ cup)

Black beans
Black-eyed peas
Butter beans
Garbanzo beans (chickpeas)
Great northern beans
Kidney beans
Lentils

Lima beans, baby
Navy beans
Peas
Pinto beans
Soybeans
Split peas
Virtually any bean or legume

Starchy Vegetables

Breadfruit *(1 serving = 1 cup)*
Corn *(1 serving = ½ cup)*
Potato *(1 serving = 1 medium)*
Sweet potato *(1 serving = 1 medium)*
Taro *(1 serving = ½ cup)*
Winter squashes *(acorn, spaghetti, butternut, etc.) (1 serving = 1 cup)*
Yam *(1 serving = 1 medium)*

Cleansing Vegetables

(Same foods as Accelerate Cycle)

Low-Sugar Fruit

(Same foods as Accelerate Cycle)

Probiotic Foods

(Same foods as Accelerate Cycle)

Friendly Fats

(Same foods as Accelerate Cycle)

Condiments

Condiments and seasonings are allowed in moderation: salsa, low-carb marinara sauce, lite soy sauce, reduced-sugar ketchup, fat-free sour cream, low-fat, low-sodium broth, Truvia (a noncaloric sweetener made from natural ingredients), sugar-free jams and jellies, vegetable cooking spray, fat-free cheeses (i.e., Parmesan), fat-free salad dressing, salt, pepper, vinegar, mustard, herbs, and spices.

Meal Planning Made Easy

On the Activate Cycle you alternate Accelerate Cycle days with Activate Cycle days. On Activate days, you eat:

- Liberal amounts of protein and cleansing vegetables
- Two daily servings of natural starches (carbohydrates)
- Two low-sugar fruit servings
- Two servings of probiotic foods
- One daily serving of friendly fat

Here's a sample menu for Cycle 2:

Wake-up drink

Every morning, as soon as you rise, drink one 8-ounce cup of hot water. Squeeze half a lemon into the cup; the lemon stimulates your digestive juices. Your goal is to drink at least six to seven more glasses of water by the end of the day.

Day 1

Breakfast

- 1 Dr. Mike's Power Cookie (see *The 17 Day Diet* for recipe)
- 1 fresh peach, sliced
- 1 cup green tea

Lunch

- Chicken salad: baked or grilled chicken breast (diced), loose-leaf lettuce, 1 sliced tomato, assorted salad veggies, 2 tablespoons olive oil mixed with 4 tablespoons balsamic vinegar
- ½ cup brown rice
- 6 ounces sugar-free fruit-flavored yogurt

Dinner

- Grilled salmon
- Steamed veggies

Snacks

- Peachy Shake (See the recipes on pages 287–294.)

The next day, Day 2, follow the Accelerate Cycle menu.

DAY 1—MY DAILY FOOD CHART   DATE

Dr. Mike's Food Tip of the Day

Shellfish—crab, clams, mussels, oysters, scallops, and shrimp—are new foods that have been added in Cycle 2 on Activate days. As long as you don't have an allergy, enjoy shellfish steamed or broiled for a low-fat, low-cholesterol, heart-healthy choice that is also a good source of protein and is full of vitamins and minerals. Shellfish also contain omega-3 fatty acids, although levels are not as high as in fatty fish like salmon and tuna.

WEIGHT

WATER INTAKE

number of 8-ounce glasses

☐ ☐ ☐ ☐
☐ ☐ ☐ ☐

FOOD INTAKE

number of servings

☐ Lean Proteins

☐ Cleansing Vegetables

☐ Natural Starch (2 servings on Activate days)

☐ Low-Sugar Fruit (2 servings)

☐ Probiotic Foods (2 servings)

☐ Friendly Fats (1–2 tablespoons)

Breakfast

_____
_____
_____
_____
_____

Lunch

_____
_____
_____
_____

Dinner

_____
_____
_____
_____

Snacks

_____
_____
_____

Dr. Mike's Workout Tip of the Day

Are your shins aching? This is a common problem for new walkers and one that can be avoided. Make sure you are increasing your speed and distance gradually. Before and after your walk, perform ankle circles and toe points as part of your stretch routine, then stretch your calves and shins after you walk. Last but not least, make sure you are wearing well-fitting walking shoes.

Cardio

DATE	ACTIVITY DESCRIPTION	DURATION	CALORIES BURNED	DISTANCE	STEPS

Toning Exercises

EXERCISES	SETS	REPS	WEIGHT	TIME	CALORIES BURNED

DAY 1—MY DAILY JOURNAL

What worked well?

_____
_____
_____

What didn't work well?

_____
_____
_____

I experienced the following challenges:

_____
_____
_____

Ways to overcome these challenges
(brainstorm as many problem-solvers as you can):

_____
_____
_____

From your list, choose the best solutions and develop
strategies for success.

_____
_____
_____

Reflections: Journal how you're feeling, your successes, anything that
comes to mind about your progress so far. Read through *The 17 Day Diet*
book to learn about all my strategies for overcoming barriers. Which
ones can you apply today?

_____
_____
_____
_____
_____
_____

DAY 2—MY DAILY FOOD CHART   DATE

Dr. Mike's Food Tip of the Day

Here's a tip for trimming all visible fat from meat: Just place it in the
freezer for 15–20 minutes, enough time for the fat to begin to harden.
Your trimming job will be much easier!

WEIGHT

WATER INTAKE

number of 8-ounce glasses

☐ ☐ ☐ ☐
☐ ☐ ☐ ☐

FOOD INTAKE

number of servings

☐ Lean Proteins

☐ Cleansing
   Vegetables

☐ Natural Starch
   (2 servings on
   Activate days)

☐ Low-Sugar Fruit
   (2 servings)

☐ Probiotic Foods
   (2 servings)

☐ Friendly Fats
   (1–2 tablespoons)

Breakfast

_____
_____
_____
_____

Lunch

_____
_____
_____
_____

Dinner

_____
_____
_____
_____

Snacks

_____
_____
_____

Dr. Mike's Workout Tip of the Day

Have you thought of purchasing a pedometer to measure your steps? Studies published in the *Journal of the American Medical Association* show people who use a pedometer (also called a step counter) are more active, lose weight, and are able to lower their blood pressure, especially if they are given a goal to increase their number of daily steps.

Cardio

DATE	ACTIVITY DESCRIPTION	DURATION	CALORIES BURNED	DISTANCE	STEPS

Toning Exercises

EXERCISES	SETS	REPS	WEIGHT	TIME	CALORIES BURNED

DAY 2—MY DAILY JOURNAL

What worked well?

_____
_____
_____

What didn't work well?

_____
_____
_____

I experienced the following challenges:

_____
_____
_____

Ways to overcome these challenges
(brainstorm as many problem-solvers as you can):

_____
_____
_____

From your list, choose the best solutions and develop
strategies for success.

_____
_____
_____

Reflections: Journal how you're feeling, your successes, anything that comes to mind about your progress so far. Read through *The 17 Day Diet* book to learn about all my strategies for overcoming barriers. Which ones can you apply today?

_____
_____
_____
_____
_____
_____

DAY 3—MY DAILY FOOD CHART   DATE

Dr. Mike's Food Tip of the Day

Some of the grains added to your food list in Cycle 2 may be new to you. Amaranth, for example, is included in the grain category but is actually a "pseudograin," making it a desirable food for those with a gluten allergy. Look for amaranth in the natural foods section of your supermarket or at a health foods store. Note: Amaranth seeds have a higher protein content than wheat!

WEIGHT

WATER INTAKE

number of 8-ounce glasses

☐ ☐ ☐ ☐
☐ ☐ ☐ ☐

FOOD INTAKE

number of servings

☐ Lean Proteins

☐ Cleansing
   Vegetables

☐ Natural Starch
   (2 servings on
   Activate days)

☐ Low-Sugar Fruit
   (2 servings)

☐ Probiotic Foods
   (2 servings)

☐ Friendly Fats
   (1–2 tablespoons)

Breakfast

_____
_____
_____
_____
_____

Lunch

_____
_____
_____
_____

Dinner

_____
_____
_____
_____

Snacks

_____
_____

Dr. Mike's Workout Tip of the Day

Got that pedometer yet? Using one can motivate you to walk more. Set a goal to walk an extra 2,000 steps per day, then check periodically to see if you need more steps for the day.

Cardio

DATE	ACTIVITY DESCRIPTION	DURATION	CALORIES BURNED	DISTANCE	STEPS

Toning Exercises

EXERCISES	SETS	REPS	WEIGHT	TIME	CALORIES BURNED

DAY 3—MY DAILY JOURNAL

What worked well?

_____
_____
_____

What didn't work well?

_____
_____
_____

I experienced the following challenges:

_____
_____
_____

Ways to overcome these challenges
(brainstorm as many problem-solvers as you can):

_____
_____
_____

From your list, choose the best solutions and develop
strategies for success.

_____
_____

Reflections: Journal how you're feeling, your successes, anything that comes to mind about your progress so far. Read through *The 17 Day Diet* book to learn about all my strategies for overcoming barriers. Which ones can you apply today?

_____
_____
_____
_____
_____
_____
_____

DAY 4—MY DAILY FOOD CHART   DATE

Dr. Mike's Food Tip of the Day

Be alert to serving sizes! What you used to consider as a serving and what a serving actually is are most likely very different things. Serving sizes for natural grains, beans/legumes, and some starchy veggies are ½ cup! Get your measuring cups out and see what half a cup looks like.

WEIGHT

WATER INTAKE

number of 8-ounce glasses

☐ ☐ ☐ ☐
☐ ☐ ☐ ☐

FOOD INTAKE
number of servings

☐ Lean Proteins

☐ Cleansing Vegetables

☐ Natural Starch (2 servings on Activate days)

☐ Low-Sugar Fruit (2 servings)

☐ Probiotic Foods (2 servings)

☐ Friendly Fats (1–2 tablespoons)

Breakfast

Lunch

Dinner

Snacks

Dr. Mike's Workout Tip of the Day

Okay, so I'm passionate about pedometers. If you're still shopping, you'll find that some pedometers just count your steps, some digital ones also measure your distance, and others estimate how many calories have been burned. Pedometers are priced to fit any budget and come with a clip or strap to attach to your waistband or belt.

Cardio

DATE	ACTIVITY DESCRIPTION	DURATION	CALORIES BURNED	DISTANCE	STEPS

Toning Exercises

EXERCISES	SETS	REPS	WEIGHT	TIME	CALORIES BURNED

DAY 4—MY DAILY JOURNAL

What worked well?

_____

_____

_____

What didn't work well?

_____

_____

_____

I experienced the following challenges:

_____

_____

_____

**Ways to overcome these challenges
(brainstorm as many problem-solvers as you can):**

_____

_____

_____

**From your list, choose the best solutions and develop
strategies for success.**

_____

_____

_____

Reflections: Journal how you're feeling, your successes, anything that comes to mind about your progress so far. Read through *The 17 Day Diet* book to learn about all my strategies for overcoming barriers. Which ones can you apply today?

_____

_____

_____

_____

_____

_____

DAY 5—MY DAILY FOOD CHART   DATE

Dr. Mike's Food Tip of the Day

Mental pictures can help you get a handle on what a serving size looks like. One cup of veggies is about the size of a baseball. Think of ½ cup of grains, legumes, or fruit as the size of half a baseball.

WEIGHT

WATER INTAKE

number of 8-ounce glasses

☐ ☐ ☐ ☐
☐ ☐ ☐ ☐

FOOD INTAKE

number of servings

☐ Lean Proteins

☐ Cleansing Vegetables

☐ Natural Starch (2 servings on Activate days)

☐ Low-Sugar Fruit (2 servings)

☐ Probiotic Foods (2 servings)

☐ Friendly Fats (1–2 tablespoons)

Breakfast

_____
_____
_____
_____
_____

Lunch

_____
_____
_____
_____
_____

Dinner

_____
_____
_____
_____
_____

Snacks

_____
_____
_____

Dr. Mike's Workout Tip of the Day

Don't just sit there! Walking at 3 mph burns about three times the calories that you burn while sitting still. At 3 mph, you can walk a mile in about 20 minutes. Up your pace to 4 mph and you'll burn five times the calories as the couch potato that you used to be!

Cardio

DATE	ACTIVITY DESCRIPTION	DURATION	CALORIES BURNED	DISTANCE	STEPS

Toning Exercises

EXERCISES	SETS	REPS	WEIGHT	TIME	CALORIES BURNED

DAY 5—MY DAILY JOURNAL

What worked well?

_____
_____
_____

What didn't work well?

_____
_____
_____

I experienced the following challenges:

_____
_____
_____

Ways to overcome these challenges
(brainstorm as many problem-solvers as you can):

_____
_____
_____

From your list, choose the best solutions and develop
strategies for success.

_____
_____
_____

Reflections: Journal how you're feeling, your successes, anything that
comes to mind about your progress so far. Read through *The 17 Day Diet*
book to learn about all my strategies for overcoming barriers. Which
ones can you apply today?

_____
_____
_____
_____
_____
_____

DAY 6—MY DAILY FOOD CHART   DATE

Dr. Mike's Food Tip of the Day

Quinoa (pronounced keen-wah) is another super-nutritious, gluten-free food that has been added in Cycle 2. Like amaranth, it is also technically a seed and is a complete protein. Found in the natural foods section of your supermarket or at a health foods store, quinoa has a slightly nutty taste and fluffy texture when boiled.

WEIGHT

WATER INTAKE

number of 8-ounce glasses

☐ ☐ ☐ ☐
☐ ☐ ☐ ☐

FOOD INTAKE

number of servings

☐ Lean Proteins

☐ Cleansing Vegetables

☐ Natural Starch (2 servings on Activate days)

☐ Low-Sugar Fruit (2 servings)

☐ Probiotic Foods (2 servings)

☐ Friendly Fats (1–2 tablespoons)

Breakfast

Lunch

Dinner

Snacks

Dr. Mike's Workout Tip of the Day

It's raining, it's too hot, it's too cold . . . These are oft-heard excuses that are just that—they are excuses! There is always going to be weather! Make sure you have a backup plan for your daily walk, like indoor mall walking, or walking on a treadmill at home or at the gym.

Cardio

DATE	ACTIVITY DESCRIPTION	DURATION	CALORIES BURNED	DISTANCE	STEPS

Toning Exercises

EXERCISES	SETS	REPS	WEIGHT	TIME	CALORIES BURNED

DAY 6—MY DAILY JOURNAL

What worked well?

_____

_____

_____

What didn't work well?

_____

_____

_____

I experienced the following challenges:

_____

_____

_____

**Ways to overcome these challenges
(brainstorm as many problem-solvers as you can):**

_____

_____

_____

**From your list, choose the best solutions and develop
strategies for success.**

_____

_____

_____

Reflections: Journal how you're feeling, your successes, anything that
comes to mind about your progress so far. Read through *The 17 Day Diet*
book to learn about all my strategies for overcoming barriers. Which
ones can you apply today?

_____

_____

_____

_____

_____

_____

DAY 7—MY DAILY FOOD CHART   DATE

Dr. Mike's Food Tip of the Day

Drinking eight 8-ounce glasses of water each day can be a challenge if you have not been used to consuming that much liquid. Try sipping water throughout the day rather than forcing down large quantities at one time. Add a lemon or lime wedge to jazz up the taste of plain water.

WEIGHT

WATER INTAKE

number of 8-ounce glasses

☐ ☐ ☐ ☐
☐ ☐ ☐ ☐

FOOD INTAKE

number of servings

☐ Lean Proteins

☐ Cleansing Vegetables

☐ Natural Starch (2 servings on Activate days)

☐ Low-Sugar Fruit (2 servings)

☐ Probiotic Foods (2 servings)

☐ Friendly Fats (1–2 tablespoons)

Breakfast
_____
_____
_____
_____
_____

Lunch
_____
_____
_____
_____

Dinner
_____
_____
_____
_____

Snacks
_____
_____
_____

Dr. Mike's Workout Tip of the Day

Which do you enjoy more? Walking alone or with others? If you are around people all day long, you may find those 17 minutes of solitude are rejuvenating and provide time for you to be alone with your thoughts. If you spend a lot of time alone, seek out a walking group or at least one other person to make your walk time a social time, too.

Cardio

DATE	ACTIVITY DESCRIPTION	DURATION	CALORIES BURNED	DISTANCE	STEPS

Toning Exercises

EXERCISES	SETS	REPS	WEIGHT	TIME	CALORIES BURNED

DAY 7—MY DAILY JOURNAL

What worked well?

_____

_____

_____

What didn't work well?

_____

_____

_____

I experienced the following challenges:

_____

_____

_____

Ways to overcome these challenges
(brainstorm as many problem-solvers as you can):

_____

_____

_____

From your list, choose the best solutions and develop
strategies for success.

_____

_____

_____

Reflections: Journal how you're feeling, your successes, anything that
comes to mind about your progress so far. Read through *The 17 Day Diet*
book to learn about all my strategies for overcoming barriers. Which
ones can you apply today?

_____

_____

_____

_____

_____

_____

_____

DAY 8—MY DAILY FOOD CHART   DATE

Dr. Mike's Food Tip of the Day

Craving pasta? Try baking spaghetti squash, a variety of winter squash having a pale yellow rind and stringy flesh that shreds into threads like thin spaghetti or vermicelli.

WEIGHT

WATER INTAKE

number of 8-ounce glasses

☐ ☐ ☐ ☐
☐ ☐ ☐ ☐

FOOD INTAKE

number of servings

☐ Lean Proteins

☐ Cleansing
   Vegetables

☐ Natural Starch
   (2 servings on
   Activate days)

☐ Low-Sugar Fruit
   (2 servings)

☐ Probiotic Foods
   (2 servings)

☐ Friendly Fats
   (1–2 tablespoons)

Breakfast

_____
_____
_____
_____
_____

Lunch

_____
_____
_____
_____
_____

Dinner

_____
_____
_____
_____

Snacks

_____
_____
_____

Dr. Mike's Workout Tip of the Day

You burn approximately 100 calories for every mile you walk. And that takes about 2,000 steps. Even though your stride will be different from someone else's, an average stride is usually about 2 to 3 feet in length. That means to complete 1 mile will take between 1,760 and 2,640 steps.

Cardio

DATE	ACTIVITY DESCRIPTION	DURATION	CALORIES BURNED	DISTANCE	STEPS

Toning Exercises

EXERCISES	SETS	REPS	WEIGHT	TIME	CALORIES BURNED

DAY 8—MY DAILY JOURNAL

What worked well?

_____
_____
_____

What didn't work well?

_____
_____
_____

I experienced the following challenges:

_____
_____
_____

**Ways to overcome these challenges
(brainstorm as many problem-solvers as you can):**

_____
_____
_____

**From your list, choose the best solutions and develop
strategies for success.**

_____
_____
_____

Reflections: Journal how you're feeling, your successes, anything that comes to mind about your progress so far. Read through *The 17 Day Diet* book to learn about all my strategies for overcoming barriers. Which ones can you apply today?

_____
_____
_____
_____
_____
_____

DAY 9—MY DAILY FOOD CHART   DATE

Dr. Mike's Food Tip of the Day

Both white and sweet potatoes are on the Cycle 2 list for the Activate Cycle and both are highly nutritious. Although sweet potatoes are slightly higher in fiber, much higher in vitamin A, and slightly higher in vitamin C, both kinds of potatoes are virtually fat-free and are very low in sodium.

WEIGHT

WATER INTAKE

number of 8-ounce glasses

☐ ☐ ☐ ☐
☐ ☐ ☐ ☐

FOOD INTAKE

number of servings

☐ Lean Proteins

☐ Cleansing Vegetables

☐ Natural Starch (2 servings on Activate days)

☐ Low-Sugar Fruit (2 servings)

☐ Probiotic Foods (2 servings)

☐ Friendly Fats (1–2 tablespoons)

Breakfast

_____
_____
_____
_____
_____

Lunch

_____
_____
_____
_____

Dinner

_____
_____
_____
_____

Snacks

_____
_____
_____

Dr. Mike's Workout Tip of the Day

If you are experience itchy legs while walking, you aren't alone. This is a common complaint among those beginning a walking program. It may be nothing more than poor circulation, which will begin to go away as you increase your activity level. Another cause may be dry skin, made worse by sweating when you exercise. In that case, moisturize before exercising and wear breathable clothing.

Cardio

DATE	ACTIVITY DESCRIPTION	DURATION	CALORIES BURNED	DISTANCE	STEPS

Toning Exercises

EXERCISES	SETS	REPS	WEIGHT	TIME	CALORIES BURNED

DAY 9—MY DAILY JOURNAL

What worked well?

_____

_____

_____

What didn't work well?

_____

_____

_____

I experienced the following challenges:

_____

_____

_____

**Ways to overcome these challenges
(brainstorm as many problem-solvers as you can):**

_____

_____

_____

**From your list, choose the best solutions and develop
strategies for success.**

_____

_____

_____

Reflections: Journal how you're feeling, your successes, anything that
comes to mind about your progress so far. Read through *The 17 Day Diet*
book to learn about all my strategies for overcoming barriers. Which
ones can you apply today?

_____

_____

_____

_____

_____

_____

_____

DAY 10—MY DAILY FOOD CHART   DATE

Dr. Mike's Food Tip of the Day

If you have always been a "meat and potatoes" kind of eater, getting used to eating vegetables may be hard for you. Make a promise to yourself that you'll try one new vegetable each week. Experiment! If you've tried cooked broccoli before and didn't like it, try it again in a raw state with a low-fat, low-calorie dip. Grilling vegetables can give them a different taste, too, especially when brushed with a low-calorie vinaigrette dressing.

WEIGHT

WATER INTAKE

number of 8-ounce glasses

☐ ☐ ☐ ☐
☐ ☐ ☐ ☐

FOOD INTAKE

number of servings

☐ Lean Proteins

☐ Cleansing Vegetables

☐ Natural Starch (2 servings on Activate days)

☐ Low-Sugar Fruit (2 servings)

☐ Probiotic Foods (2 servings)

☐ Friendly Fats (1–2 tablespoons)

Breakfast

Lunch

Dinner

Snacks

Dr. Mike's Workout Tip of the Day

It's a heart thing! You may be a loving friend and partner, but without regular exercise, you are not being a friend to your heart. Love yourself enough to do all you can to keep your heart pumping efficiently. Walking does just that, along with improving breathing and blood flow, and lowering high blood pressure and cholesterol.

Cardio

DATE	ACTIVITY DESCRIPTION	DURATION	CALORIES BURNED	DISTANCE	STEPS

Toning Exercises

EXERCISES	SETS	REPS	WEIGHT	TIME	CALORIES BURNED

DAY 10—MY DAILY JOURNAL

What worked well?

_____
_____
_____

What didn't work well?

_____
_____
_____

I experienced the following challenges:

_____
_____
_____

Ways to overcome these challenges
(brainstorm as many problem-solvers as you can):

_____
_____
_____

From your list, choose the best solutions and develop
strategies for success.

_____
_____
_____

Reflections: Journal how you're feeling, your successes, anything that comes to mind about your progress so far. Read through *The 17 Day Diet* book to learn about all my strategies for overcoming barriers. Which ones can you apply today?

_____
_____
_____
_____
_____
_____

DAY 11—MY DAILY FOOD CHART   DATE

Dr. Mike's Food Tip of the Day

While green tea is a recommended beverage (3 cups a day) due to the natural chemicals it contains that increase fat-burning and stimulate calorie-burning, it can be an acquired taste. The good news is that green tea varieties with other flavors added—mint, lemon, jasmine, pomegranate, mango, peach, and orange—are readily available and may tempt you to drink more of it.

WEIGHT

WATER INTAKE

number of 8-ounce glasses

☐ ☐ ☐ ☐
☐ ☐ ☐ ☐

FOOD INTAKE

number of servings

☐ Lean Proteins

☐ Cleansing Vegetables

☐ Natural Starch (2 servings on Activate days)

☐ Low-Sugar Fruit (2 servings)

☐ Probiotic Foods (2 servings)

☐ Friendly Fats (1–2 tablespoons)

Breakfast

Lunch

Dinner

Snacks

Dr. Mike's Workout Tip of the Day

Get moving together! Families that exercise together find they become closer and their relationships improve. If you are an overweight parent, exercising with your spouse and kids can help to change the family dynamic as you begin to lead by example.

Cardio

DATE	ACTIVITY DESCRIPTION	DURATION	CALORIES BURNED	DISTANCE	STEPS

Toning Exercises

EXERCISES	SETS	REPS	WEIGHT	TIME	CALORIES BURNED

DAY 11—MY DAILY JOURNAL

What worked well?

_____
_____
_____

What didn't work well?

_____
_____
_____

I experienced the following challenges:

_____
_____
_____

**Ways to overcome these challenges
(brainstorm as many problem-solvers as you can):**

_____
_____
_____

**From your list, choose the best solutions and develop
strategies for success.**

_____
_____
_____

Reflections: Journal how you're feeling, your successes, anything that
comes to mind about your progress so far. Read through *The 17 Day Diet*
book to learn about all my strategies for overcoming barriers. Which
ones can you apply today?

_____
_____
_____
_____
_____
_____

DAY 12—MY DAILY FOOD CHART   DATE

Dr. Mike's Food Tip of the Day

Feeling full and feeling fine! On the Activate days of Cycle 2, you're eating two servings of starchy carbs, but they are the natural, slow-digesting kind. Oatmeal, whole grains, brown rice, beans, legumes, and potatoes are all in this category. They take a long time to digest and keep you feeling full and satisfied.

WEIGHT

WATER INTAKE

number of 8-ounce glasses

☐ ☐ ☐ ☐
☐ ☐ ☐ ☐

FOOD INTAKE

number of servings

☐ Lean Proteins

☐ Cleansing Vegetables

☐ Natural Starch (2 servings on Activate days)

☐ Low-Sugar Fruit (2 servings)

☐ Probiotic Foods (2 servings)

☐ Friendly Fats (1–2 tablespoons)

Breakfast

_____
_____
_____
_____

Lunch

_____
_____
_____
_____

Dinner

_____
_____
_____
_____

Snacks

_____
_____
_____

Dr. Mike's Workout Tip of the Day

I can feel it in my bones . . . Are you over 35? If so, you are already beginning to lose bone density, which can eventually lead to osteoporosis. The good news is that exercise preserves bone density and can actually build bone in older adults, while a sedentary lifestyle causes a rapid loss of bone density.

Cardio

DATE	ACTIVITY DESCRIPTION	DURATION	CALORIES BURNED	DISTANCE	STEPS

Toning Exercises

EXERCISES	SETS	REPS	WEIGHT	TIME	CALORIES BURNED

DAY 12—MY DAILY JOURNAL

What worked well?

_____
_____
_____

What didn't work well?

_____
_____
_____

I experienced the following challenges:

_____
_____
_____

**Ways to overcome these challenges
(brainstorm as many problem-solvers as you can):**

_____
_____
_____

**From your list, choose the best solutions and develop
strategies for success.**

_____
_____
_____

Reflections: Journal how you're feeling, your successes, anything that
comes to mind about your progress so far. Read through *The 17 Day Diet*
book to learn about all my strategies for overcoming barriers. Which
ones can you apply today?

_____
_____
_____
_____
_____
_____

DAY 13—MY DAILY FOOD CHART   DATE

Dr. Mike's Food Tip of the Day

I included my Hunger/Fullness Meter in *The 17 Day Diet* book to help you gauge your hunger and fullness. Rating your hunger from being "a little hungry" to "stomach growling hungry" can mean the difference between success and failure. Don't let yourself get too hungry! There is no reason to get there. By the same token, don't let your fullness meter get to the "stuffed" stage! Learn to stop eating when you're not quite full.

WEIGHT

WATER INTAKE

number of 8-ounce glasses

☐ ☐ ☐ ☐
☐ ☐ ☐ ☐

FOOD INTAKE

number of servings

☐ Lean Proteins

☐ Cleansing Vegetables

☐ Natural Starch (2 servings on Activate days)

☐ Low-Sugar Fruit (2 servings)

☐ Probiotic Foods (2 servings)

☐ Friendly Fats (1–2 tablespoons)

Breakfast

Lunch

Dinner

Snacks

Dr. Mike's Workout Tip of the Day

Are you engaging in at least 17 minutes of daily exercise since Day 1 (of Cycle 1) of the 17 Day Diet? That means you have now been exercising for a total of 30 days! Bravo! If we were to check your cholesterol today, your LDL (bad) cholesterol level should have fallen by nearly 30 percent—similar to the decrease seen with some cholesterol-lowering drugs!

Cardio

DATE	ACTIVITY DESCRIPTION	DURATION	CALORIES BURNED	DISTANCE	STEPS

Toning Exercises

EXERCISES	SETS	REPS	WEIGHT	TIME	CALORIES BURNED

DAY 13—MY DAILY JOURNAL

What worked well?

_____

_____

_____

What didn't work well?

_____

_____

_____

I experienced the following challenges:

_____

_____

_____

**Ways to overcome these challenges
(brainstorm as many problem-solvers as you can):**

_____

_____

_____

**From your list, choose the best solutions and develop
strategies for success.**

_____

_____

_____

Reflections: Journal how you're feeling, your successes, anything that
comes to mind about your progress so far. Read through *The 17 Day Diet*
book to learn about all my strategies for overcoming barriers. Which
ones can you apply today?

_____

_____

_____

_____

_____

_____

_____

DAY 14—MY DAILY FOOD CHART   DATE

Dr. Mike's Food Tip of the Day

High-fructose corn syrup (HFCS), found in soft drinks, meats, cheeses, and many other foods, should be limited, along with all other added sweeteners, whenever possible. Get used to checking labels for ingredients. As obesity has risen in our nation, so has consumption of HFCS. It quickly turns into body fat and can cause the body to overproduce insulin, which could lead to type 2 diabetes.

WEIGHT

WATER INTAKE

number of 8-ounce glasses

☐ ☐ ☐ ☐
☐ ☐ ☐ ☐

FOOD INTAKE

number of servings

☐ Lean Proteins

☐ Cleansing Vegetables

☐ Natural Starch (2 servings on Activate days)

☐ Low-Sugar Fruit (2 servings)

☐ Probiotic Foods (2 servings)

☐ Friendly Fats (1–2 tablespoons)

Breakfast

Lunch

Dinner

Snacks

Dr. Mike's Workout Tip of the Day

Shake it up! After a while, you may become bored with doing the same thing day after day. Even if you enjoy walking, you may need to change your route, the time of day you walk, or the entire surroundings of your walk. Drive to a local park or visit the botanical gardens or the zoo to get plenty of exercise while stimulating your senses with the beauty around you.

Cardio

DATE	ACTIVITY DESCRIPTION	DURATION	CALORIES BURNED	DISTANCE	STEPS

Toning Exercises

EXERCISES	SETS	REPS	WEIGHT	TIME	CALORIES BURNED

DAY 14—MY DAILY JOURNAL

What worked well?

_____
_____
_____

What didn't work well?

_____
_____
_____

I experienced the following challenges:

_____
_____
_____

Ways to overcome these challenges
(brainstorm as many problem-solvers as you can):

_____
_____
_____

From your list, choose the best solutions and develop
strategies for success.

_____
_____
_____

Reflections: Journal how you're feeling, your successes, anything that
comes to mind about your progress so far. Read through *The 17 Day Diet*
book to learn about all my strategies for overcoming barriers. Which
ones can you apply today?

_____
_____
_____
_____
_____
_____

DAY 15—MY DAILY FOOD CHART   DATE

Dr. Mike's Food Tip of the Day

Visualize a particular food superglued to your rear, hips, or tummy. Now imagine how gross it's going to taste with superglue on it. Until superglue comes in new flavors, this should work to keep you away from fattening goodies.

WEIGHT

WATER INTAKE

number of 8-ounce glasses

☐ ☐ ☐ ☐
☐ ☐ ☐ ☐

FOOD INTAKE

number of servings

☐ Lean Proteins

☐ Cleansing Vegetables

☐ Natural Starch (2 servings on Activate days)

☐ Low-Sugar Fruit (2 servings)

☐ Probiotic Foods (2 servings)

☐ Friendly Fats (1–2 tablespoons)

Breakfast

_____
_____
_____
_____
_____

Lunch

_____
_____
_____
_____

Dinner

_____
_____
_____
_____

Snacks

_____
_____
_____

Dr. Mike's Workout Tip of the Day

Before you skip your workout, ask yourself: Will I regret it later? Think about how you'll feel when you get into bed tonight knowing you have let yourself down by not taking at least 17 minutes out of your day to move your body! Instead, think about how you'll feel about yourself after you live up to your commitment to exercise daily.

Cardio

DATE	ACTIVITY DESCRIPTION	DURATION	CALORIES BURNED	DISTANCE	STEPS

Toning Exercises

EXERCISES	SETS	REPS	WEIGHT	TIME	CALORIES BURNED

DAY 15—MY DAILY JOURNAL

What worked well?

_____

_____

_____

What didn't work well?

_____

_____

_____

I experienced the following challenges:

_____

_____

_____

Ways to overcome these challenges
(brainstorm as many problem-solvers as you can):

_____

_____

_____

From your list, choose the best solutions and develop
strategies for success.

_____

_____

_____

Reflections: Journal how you're feeling, your successes, anything that
comes to mind about your progress so far. Read through *The 17 Day Diet*
book to learn about all my strategies for overcoming barriers. Which
ones can you apply today?

_____

_____

_____

_____

_____

_____

_____

DAY 16—MY DAILY FOOD CHART   DATE

Dr. Mike's Food Tip of the Day

How are you enjoying your wake-up drink—an 8-ounce cup of hot water with half a lemon squeezed into it? Not only is it the first of the 8 glasses of water you are to drink by the end of the day, but it stimulates your digestive juices and rehydrates your body after a night's sleep so you can properly absorb nutrients from the food you'll eat throughout the day. Now, go ahead and enjoy a cup of green tea, or if you must, that cup of coffee!

WEIGHT

WATER INTAKE

number of 8-ounce glasses

☐ ☐ ☐ ☐
☐ ☐ ☐ ☐

FOOD INTAKE

number of servings

☐ Lean Proteins

☐ Cleansing Vegetables

☐ Natural Starch (2 servings on Activate days)

☐ Low-Sugar Fruit (2 servings)

☐ Probiotic Foods (2 servings)

☐ Friendly Fats (1–2 tablespoons)

Breakfast

Lunch

Dinner

Snacks

Dr. Mike's Workout Tip of the Day

Use the talk test: If you aren't sure you are walking fast enough to increase your heart rate and your fitness level, take the talk test. If you can sing along with that favorite song you're listening to on your iPod, you are walking too slowly. If you can't carry on a simple conversation with your walking buddy and are gasping for breath as you walk, you are walking too fast.

Cardio

DATE	ACTIVITY DESCRIPTION	DURATION	CALORIES BURNED	DISTANCE	STEPS

Toning Exercises

EXERCISES	SETS	REPS	WEIGHT	TIME	CALORIES BURNED

DAY 16—MY DAILY JOURNAL

What worked well?

_____

_____

_____

What didn't work well?

_____

_____

_____

I experienced the following challenges:

_____

_____

_____

Ways to overcome these challenges
(brainstorm as many problem-solvers as you can):

_____

_____

_____

From your list, choose the best solutions and develop
strategies for success.

_____

_____

_____

Reflections: Journal how you're feeling, your successes, anything that
comes to mind about your progress so far. Read through *The 17 Day Diet*
book to learn about all my strategies for overcoming barriers. Which
ones can you apply today?

_____

_____

_____

_____

_____

_____

DAY 17—MY DAILY FOOD CHART   DATE

Dr. Mike's Food Tip of the Day

Just like us, the parts of the animal that are the leanest are those that get the most exercise. When choosing lean cuts of meat, remember that they may need to be tenderized to keep them moist and flavorful. Marinating meats in fat-free broth, fat-free salad dressings, wine, or fruit juice can transform a lean cut of meat from tough to tasty!

WEIGHT

WATER INTAKE

number of 8-ounce glasses
☐ ☐ ☐ ☐
☐ ☐ ☐ ☐

FOOD INTAKE

number of servings

☐ Lean Proteins

☐ Cleansing
   Vegetables

☐ Natural Starch
   (2 servings on
   Activate days)

☐ Low-Sugar Fruit
   (2 servings)

☐ Probiotic Foods
   (2 servings)

☐ Friendly Fats
   (1–2 tablespoons)

Breakfast

_____
_____
_____
_____
_____

Lunch

_____
_____
_____
_____

Dinner

_____
_____
_____
_____

Snacks

_____
_____
_____

Dr. Mike's Workout Tip of the Day

Men and women who weigh the same amount burn approximately the same number of calories if they complete the same activity. But in so many ways, men and women's exercise preferences differ. Men tend to shy away from the group exercise classes, for example. Do what you love, and the results will follow.

Cardio

DATE	ACTIVITY DESCRIPTION	DURATION	CALORIES BURNED	DISTANCE	STEPS

Toning Exercises

EXERCISES	SETS	REPS	WEIGHT	TIME	CALORIES BURNED

DAY 17—MY DAILY JOURNAL

What worked well?

_____
_____
_____

What didn't work well?

_____
_____
_____

I experienced the following challenges:

_____
_____
_____

**Ways to overcome these challenges
(brainstorm as many problem-solvers as you can):**

_____
_____
_____

**From your list, choose the best solutions and develop
strategies for success.**

_____
_____
_____

Reflections: Journal how you're feeling, your successes, anything that
comes to mind about your progress so far. Read through *The 17 Day Diet*
book to learn about all my strategies for overcoming barriers. Which
ones can you apply today?

_____
_____
_____
_____
_____
_____
_____

Review: Weight-Loss Checklist—Cycle 2

••

It is only natural that you may experience obstacles as you move through each cycle of the 17 Day Diet. Ask yourself whether you may be sabotaging your success by getting off track in one of these ways:

1. Am I skipping meals, then overeating later in the day?

    ☐ **Always**   ☐ **Sometimes**   ☐ **Rarely or Never**

2. Am I taking second helpings?

    ☐ **Always**   ☐ **Sometimes**   ☐ **Rarely or Never**

3. Am I failing to plan my meals in advance or to stick to my plan?

    ☐ **Always**   ☐ **Sometimes**   ☐ **Rarely or Never**

4. Am I watching television while eating?

    ☐ **Always**   ☐ **Sometimes**   ☐ **Rarely or Never**

5. Am I letting other things distract me from working out every day?

    ☐ **Always**   ☐ **Sometimes**   ☐ **Rarely or Never**

My top areas to work on in the next cycle:

_____

_____

_____

_____

I lost _____ pounds on Cycle 2.

How do you feel about your weight loss so far?

_____

_____

_____

_____

CYCLE 3

. . . .

Achieve

GOAL

To develop good eating habits through the reintroduction of additional foods and move you closer to your goal weight.

What to Eat: The Achieve Cycle Expanded Food List

Where indicated, add foods to your diet in addition to those you ate on the first two cycles.

Proteins

(1 serving = 4 to 6 ounces, or the amount that can fit in the palm of your hand)

Fish and shellfish *(from Accelerate and Activate lists)*

Lean meats *(from Accelerate and Activate lists)*

Poultry *(from Accelerate and Activate lists, including eggs and egg whites)*

Additional proteins:

Canadian bacon

Cornish hen

Pheasant

Quail

Reduced-fat turkey bacon, sausage, or lunch meat

Natural Starches

Breads (1 slice = 1 serving)

Cracked wheat

Fiber-enriched bread

Gluten-free bread

Multigrain bread

Oat bran bread

Pumpernickel

Rye bread

Sugar-free bread

Whole-grain bagel *(½ = 1 serving)*

Whole-wheat pita bread, 1 pocket

Whole-wheat tortilla, 10 inch

High-Fiber Cereals (1 cup = 1 serving, unless where indicated)

Kellogg's All-Bran

Kellogg's All-Bran Bran Buds

Fiber One

Gluten-free cold cereals

Low-sugar granola *(½ cup = 1 serving)*

Pasta (½ cup = 1 serving)

Whole-wheat pasta

Gluten-free pasta

Vegetable-based pasta

High-fiber pasta

Shirataki pasta *(a very low-calorie pasta made from tofu and sweet potatoes—1 cup = 1 serving)*

Vegetables—Unlimited

All cleansing vegetables

Alfalfa

Broccoli sprouts

Chilis

Cilantro

Fennel

Grape leaves

Jicama

Kelp and other edible seaweeds

Kohlrabi

Peapods

Radishes

Rhubarb

Rutabaga

Summer squash

Swiss chard

Yellow wax beans

Zucchini
Virtually any vegetable

Fruits—2 servings daily

(1 serving = 1 piece or 1 cup chopped fresh fruit)

Apricots
Bananas
Cherries
Currants
Figs
Guava
Kiwi
Kumquats
Mango
Nopales *(edible cactus)*
Papaya
Pineapple
Pomegranate
Tangelo
Tangerine
Virtually any fresh fruit

Note: If you are watching your sugar intake, stick to lower sugar fruits. These include apples, berries (all varieties), cherries, grapefruit, orange, peach, pear, and plum

Probiotics, Dairy, and Dairy Substitutes: 1 to 2 servings daily

Note: Some people don't like dairy foods or can't digest them properly. If you're one of them, try dairy substitutes instead (see below). Try to eat at least one serving daily from this list while on the Achieve Cycle.

Probiotic foods from Accelerate and Activate Cycles
Low-calorie cheeses (brie, camembert, fontina, low-fat cheddar,
    edam, feta, goat, limburger, and part-skim mozzarella)
    (2 ounces = 1 serving)

Low-fat cottage cheese *(½ cup = 1 serving)*
Low-fat milk, including skim *(1 cup = 1 serving)*
Low-fat ricotta cheese *(½ cup = 1 serving)*
Dairy substitutes: Sugar-free rice, almond, or soy milk *(1 cup = 1 serving)*

Friendly Fats—1 to 2 tablespoons daily, unless where indicated

Avocado *(¼ fruit = 1 serving)*
Canola oil *(1 tablespoon = 1 serving)*
Light mayonnaise *(2 tablespoons = 1 serving)*
Mayonnaise *(1 tablespoon = 1 serving)*
Nuts or seeds, unoiled *(2 tablespoons = 1 serving)*
Reduced-calorie margarines *(2 tablespoons = 1 serving)*
Reduced-fat salad dressings *(2 tablespoons = 1 serving)*
Salad dressings *(1 tablespoon = 1 serving)*
Trans-free margarines *(1 tablespoon = 1 serving)*
Walnut oil *(1 tablespoon = 1 serving)*

Optional Snacks

These snacks are all under 100 calories. Plus, they're filling and fun to eat.

Babybel low-fat cheese—2 disks
Frozen fruit bar
Fudgsicle, 100 Calorie bar
Granola bar, reduced sugar and fat
Microwave popcorn, light *(4 cups)*
Skinny Cow ice cream sandwich
String cheese—1 stick
Sugar-free pudding cup

Meal Planning Made Easy

Each day, for the next 17 days, you'll eat:

- Controlled portions of protein from an expanded list (1 serving = 4 to 6 ounces, or roughly the amount that can fit in the palm of your hand).
- Liberal amounts of vegetables from an expanded list.
- Two servings of natural starches, high-fiber cereals, or pasta from an expanded list.
- Two servings of fruit from an expanded list.
- One to two servings from probiotics, low-fat dairy, or dairy substitutes.
- One serving of fat from an expanded list.
- Optional snacks.
- Optional daily serving of alcohol.

Here is a sample menu on the Achieve Cycle:

Wake-up drink

Every morning, as soon as you rise, drink one 8-ounce cup of hot water. Squeeze half a lemon into the cup; the lemon stimulates your digestive juices. Your goal is to drink at least six to seven more glasses of water by the end of the day.

Day 1

Breakfast

- 1 slice whole-wheat toast
- 1 poached, soft-boiled, or hard-boiled egg
- ½ grapefruit
- 1 cup green tea

Lunch

- Chicken Caesar salad: 4 to 6 ounces grilled chicken breast, cut into pieces; 2 cups romaine lettuce; other desired salad veggies; 2 tablespoons light Caesar dressing
- 1 slice whole-wheat toast
- 1 serving fresh fruit
- 1 cup green tea

Dinner

- 4 to 6 ounces roasted pork tenderloin
- 1 to 2 cups tossed mixed salad with 2 tablespoons fat-free dressing
- 1 cup green tea

Snacks

- 1 probiotic, dairy, or dairy substitute serving
- 1 frozen fruit bar

DAY 1—MY DAILY FOOD CHART   DATE

Dr. Mike's Food Tip of the Day

Remember that protein portions in Cycle 3 are to be limited to about the size of a kitchen sponge, a deck of cards, or the palm of your hand (3–4 ounces). Having a visual picture in mind helps you achieve good eating habits for a lifetime, including portion control.

WEIGHT

WATER INTAKE

number of 8-ounce glasses

☐ ☐ ☐ ☐
☐ ☐ ☐ ☐

FOOD INTAKE
number of servings

☐ Lean Proteins

☐ Cleansing
   Vegetables

☐ Natural Starch/
   High-Fiber
   Cereal/or Pasta
   (2 servings)

☐ Fruit
   (2 servings)

☐ Probiotic Foods/
   Dairy/Dairy Subs
   (1–2 servings)

☐ Friendly Fats
   (1–2 tablespoons)

☐ Optional Snack

Breakfast

_____
_____
_____
_____
_____

Lunch

_____
_____
_____
_____

Dinner

_____
_____
_____
_____

Snacks

_____
_____

Dr. Mike's Workout Tip of the Day

Congratulations! You've made it to Cycle 3. It's time to ramp up your aerobic exercise! If you want to speed up your weight loss during this cycle, strive to do 45 to 60 minutes of aerobic exercise as many days of the week as you can.

Cardio

DATE	ACTIVITY DESCRIPTION	DURATION	CALORIES BURNED	DISTANCE	STEPS

Toning Exercises

EXERCISES	SETS	REPS	WEIGHT	TIME	CALORIES BURNED

DAY 1—MY DAILY JOURNAL

What worked well?

_____

_____

_____

What didn't work well?

_____

_____

_____

I experienced the following challenges:

_____

_____

_____

Ways to overcome these challenges
(brainstorm as many problem-solvers as you can):

_____

_____

_____

From your list, choose the best solutions and develop
strategies for success.

_____

_____

_____

Reflections: Journal how you're feeling, your successes, anything that comes to mind about your progress so far. Read through *The 17 Day Diet* book to learn about all my strategies for overcoming barriers. Which ones can you apply today?

_____

_____

_____

_____

_____

_____

_____

DAY 2—MY DAILY FOOD CHART   DATE

Dr. Mike's Food Tip of the Day

One of the additional poultry choices in Cycle 3 is Cornish hen, a type of domestic chicken that averages between 1 and 1½ pounds. Half a hen cooked with skin removed is 150 calories and 5 grams of fat. With skin, half a hen is 340 calories and a whopping 25 grams of fat! That's why removing skin from all poultry is necessary on the 17 Day Diet.

WEIGHT

WATER INTAKE

number of 8-ounce glasses

☐ ☐ ☐ ☐
☐ ☐ ☐ ☐

FOOD INTAKE

number of servings

☐ Lean Proteins

☐ Cleansing Vegetables

☐ Natural Starch/ High-Fiber Cereal/or Pasta (2 servings)

☐ Fruit (2 servings)

☐ Probiotic Foods/ Dairy/Dairy Subs (1–2 servings)

☐ Friendly Fats (1–2 tablespoons)

☐ Optional Snack

Breakfast

Lunch

Dinner

Snacks

Dr. Mike's Workout Tip of the Day

Aerobics is defined as using the same large muscle group, rhythmically, for a period of 15 to 20 minutes or longer while maintaining 60–80 percent of your maximum heart rate. Any type of aerobic exercise—walking, running, biking, swimming, tennis, or whatever—can be used to speed up weight loss by creating a calorie deficit: burning more calories than you take in.

Cardio

DATE	ACTIVITY DESCRIPTION	DURATION	CALORIES BURNED	DISTANCE	STEPS

Toning Exercises

EXERCISES	SETS	REPS	WEIGHT	TIME	CALORIES BURNED

DAY 2—MY DAILY JOURNAL

What worked well?

_____

_____

_____

What didn't work well?

_____

_____

_____

I experienced the following challenges:

_____

_____

_____

Ways to overcome these challenges
(brainstorm as many problem-solvers as you can):

_____

_____

_____

From your list, choose the best solutions and develop
strategies for success.

_____

_____

_____

Reflections: Journal how you're feeling, your successes, anything that
comes to mind about your progress so far. Read through *The 17 Day Diet*
book to learn about all my strategies for overcoming barriers. Which
ones can you apply today?

_____

_____

_____

_____

_____

_____

DAY 3—MY DAILY FOOD CHART   DATE

Dr. Mike's Food Tip of the Day

If you've ever had an Egg McMuffin from McDonald's, you've had Canadian bacon—another new protein choice added in Cycle 3. Canadian bacon is a pork product that looks and tastes more like ham than bacon. Try making your own low-fat version of an Egg McMuffin with Canadian bacon (45 calories, 2 grams fat per slice).

WEIGHT

WATER INTAKE

number of 8-ounce glasses

☐ ☐ ☐ ☐
☐ ☐ ☐ ☐

FOOD INTAKE

number of servings

☐ Lean Proteins

☐ Cleansing
Vegetables

☐ Natural Starch/
High-Fiber
Cereal/or Pasta
(2 servings)

☐ Fruit
(2 servings)

☐ Probiotic Foods/
Dairy/Dairy Subs
(1–2 servings)

☐ Friendly Fats
(1–2 tablespoons)

☐ Optional Snack

Breakfast

Lunch

Dinner

Snacks

Dr. Mike's Workout Tip of the Day

Low-impact aerobic activities are best for those with knee problems, as they help tone leg muscles supporting the knee joint that absorb the shock placed on the knee. There are lots of low-impact choices, including walking, swimming, water aerobics, low-impact aerobic dance classes, stationary bike riding, and elliptical training.

Cardio

DATE	ACTIVITY DESCRIPTION	DURATION	CALORIES BURNED	DISTANCE	STEPS

Toning Exercises

EXERCISES	SETS	REPS	WEIGHT	TIME	CALORIES BURNED

DAY 3—MY DAILY JOURNAL

What worked well?

_____
_____
_____

What didn't work well?

_____
_____
_____

I experienced the following challenges:

_____
_____
_____

Ways to overcome these challenges
(brainstorm as many problem-solvers as you can):

_____
_____
_____

From your list, choose the best solutions and develop
strategies for success.

_____
_____
_____

Reflections: Journal how you're feeling, your successes, anything that
comes to mind about your progress so far. Read through *The 17 Day Diet*
book to learn about all my strategies for overcoming barriers. Which
ones can you apply today?

_____
_____
_____
_____
_____
_____
_____

DAY 4—MY DAILY FOOD CHART   DATE

Dr. Mike's Food Tip of the Day

Who's up for popcorn and a movie? In Cycle 3, you can enjoy a snack of up to 4 cups of light microwave popcorn. Popcorn is a highly nutritious whole grain that is low calorie (without butter) and contains 40 or more nutrients. It has more protein than any other cereal grain, is iron rich, and is high in fiber.

WEIGHT

WATER INTAKE

number of 8-ounce glasses

☐ ☐ ☐ ☐
☐ ☐ ☐ ☐

FOOD INTAKE

number of servings

☐ Lean Proteins

☐ Cleansing Vegetables

☐ Natural Starch/ High-Fiber Cereal/or Pasta (2 servings)

☐ Fruit (2 servings)

☐ Probiotic Foods/ Dairy/Dairy Subs (1–2 servings)

☐ Friendly Fats (1–2 tablespoons)

☐ Optional Snack

Breakfast

_____
_____
_____
_____
_____

Lunch

_____
_____
_____

Dinner

_____
_____
_____
_____

Snacks

_____
_____

Dr. Mike's Workout Tip of the Day

Do all you can to avoid exercise injuries! Make sure you have well-fitting shoes especially made for aerobics or cross-training. You need a shoe with lateral support for side-to-side movements, cushioning to absorb impact, and proper arch support.

Cardio

DATE	ACTIVITY DESCRIPTION	DURATION	CALORIES BURNED	DISTANCE	STEPS

Toning Exercises

EXERCISES	SETS	REPS	WEIGHT	TIME	CALORIES BURNED

DAY 4—MY DAILY JOURNAL

What worked well?

_____
_____
_____

What didn't work well?

_____
_____
_____

I experienced the following challenges:

_____
_____
_____

Ways to overcome these challenges
(brainstorm as many problem-solvers as you can):

_____
_____
_____

From your list, choose the best solutions and develop
strategies for success.

_____
_____
_____

Reflections: Journal how you're feeling, your successes, anything that
comes to mind about your progress so far. Read through *The 17 Day Diet*
book to learn about all my strategies for overcoming barriers. Which
ones can you apply today?

_____
_____
_____
_____
_____
_____

DAY 5—MY DAILY FOOD CHART   DATE

Dr. Mike's Food Tip of the Day

One and only one . . . alcoholic drink, that is. That's a new freedom you've been given in Cycle 3, but portion control applies here, too. If you choose to incorporate one glass of wine into your daily diet, that means 5 ounces, not half the bottle! Here's a tip: First pour 5 ounces of water into your wineglass. Then you'll know what 5 ounces looks like!

WEIGHT

WATER INTAKE

number of 8-ounce glasses

☐ ☐ ☐ ☐
☐ ☐ ☐ ☐

FOOD INTAKE

number of servings

☐ Lean Proteins

☐ Cleansing Vegetables

☐ Natural Starch/ High-Fiber Cereal/or Pasta (2 servings)

☐ Fruit (2 servings)

☐ Probiotic Foods/ Dairy/Dairy Subs (1–2 servings)

☐ Friendly Fats (1–2 tablespoons)

☐ Optional Snack

Breakfast

Lunch

Dinner

Snacks

Dr. Mike's Workout Tip of the Day

If you are walking or jogging outdoors, you are most likely "pounding the pavement" on concrete, a hard surface that can cause stress injuries like shin splints or tendinitis. But good shoes can help. Walking and jogging on dirt paths or grass is softer, but there can be holes and uneven surfaces to trip you up, so just be careful out there!

Cardio

DATE	ACTIVITY DESCRIPTION	DURATION	CALORIES BURNED	DISTANCE	STEPS

Toning Exercises

EXERCISES	SETS	REPS	WEIGHT	TIME	CALORIES BURNED

DAY 5—MY DAILY JOURNAL

What worked well?

_____

_____

_____

What didn't work well?

_____

_____

_____

I experienced the following challenges:

_____

_____

_____

Ways to overcome these challenges
(brainstorm as many problem-solvers as you can):

_____

_____

_____

From your list, choose the best solutions and develop
strategies for success.

_____

_____

_____

Reflections: Journal how you're feeling, your successes, anything that
comes to mind about your progress so far. Read through *The 17 Day Diet*
book to learn about all my strategies for overcoming barriers. Which
ones can you apply today?

_____

_____

_____

_____

_____

_____

DAY 6—MY DAILY FOOD CHART   DATE

Dr. Mike's Food Tip of the Day

Ah, pasta! Have you been missing it? Combine pasta with nutrient-dense foods, including high-fiber vegetables, beans, fish, poultry, and lean meats for a highly nutritious and satisfying meal. Make sure the pasta you choose is whole wheat, high fiber, vegetable based, or gluten free.

WEIGHT

WATER INTAKE

number of 8-ounce glasses

☐ ☐ ☐ ☐
☐ ☐ ☐ ☐

FOOD INTAKE

number of servings

☐ Lean Proteins

☐ Cleansing Vegetables

☐ Natural Starch/ High-Fiber Cereal/or Pasta (2 servings)

☐ Fruit (2 servings)

☐ Probiotic Foods/ Dairy/Dairy Subs (1–2 servings)

☐ Friendly Fats (1–2 tablespoons)

☐ Optional Snack

Breakfast

_____
_____
_____
_____

Lunch

_____
_____
_____
_____

Dinner

_____
_____
_____

Snacks

_____
_____

Dr. Mike's Workout Tip of the Day

Avoid the soreness and pain that can be caused by overuse of your muscles by always starting with a few minutes of warm-up exercises and ending with a cooldown and a final stretch. A warm bath or shower and a foot soak with Epsom salts will also help to prevent any possible soreness.

Cardio

DATE	ACTIVITY DESCRIPTION	DURATION	CALORIES BURNED	DISTANCE	STEPS

Toning Exercises

EXERCISES	SETS	REPS	WEIGHT	TIME	CALORIES BURNED

DAY 6—MY DAILY JOURNAL

What worked well?

_____
_____
_____

What didn't work well?

_____
_____
_____

I experienced the following challenges:

_____
_____
_____

**Ways to overcome these challenges
(brainstorm as many problem-solvers as you can):**

_____
_____
_____

**From your list, choose the best solutions and develop
strategies for success.**

_____
_____
_____

Reflections: Journal how you're feeling, your successes, anything that
comes to mind about your progress so far. Read through *The 17 Day Diet*
book to learn about all my strategies for overcoming barriers. Which
ones can you apply today?

_____
_____
_____
_____
_____
_____

DAY 7—MY DAILY FOOD CHART   DATE

Dr. Mike's Food Tip of the Day

If you haven't tried udon noodles, a low-fat, cholesterol-free Japanese pan noodle made from wheat flour, put them on your shopping list for next week. Udon noodles are a great addition to a stir-fry dish or Asian soup, and can even be served cold as a salad ingredient.

WEIGHT

WATER INTAKE

number of 8-ounce glasses

☐ ☐ ☐ ☐
☐ ☐ ☐ ☐

FOOD INTAKE

number of servings

☐ Lean Proteins

☐ Cleansing Vegetables

☐ Natural Starch/ High-Fiber Cereal/or Pasta (2 servings)

☐ Fruit (2 servings)

☐ Probiotic Foods/ Dairy/Dairy Subs (1–2 servings)

☐ Friendly Fats (1–2 tablespoons)

☐ Optional Snack

Breakfast

Lunch

Dinner

Snacks

Dr. Mike's Workout Tip of the Day

Is it best to exercise in the morning or the evening? There is no bad time to exercise, as long as it is a time that works for you! If you have an early morning meeting, just make sure to schedule your workout over your lunch hour or after your workday has ended. Make your workout a priority, and not something that can be canceled or rescheduled to another day.

Cardio

DATE	ACTIVITY DESCRIPTION	DURATION	CALORIES BURNED	DISTANCE	STEPS

Toning Exercises

EXERCISES	SETS	REPS	WEIGHT	TIME	CALORIES BURNED

DAY 7—MY DAILY JOURNAL

What worked well?

_____

_____

_____

What didn't work well?

_____

_____

_____

I experienced the following challenges:

_____

_____

_____

Ways to overcome these challenges
(brainstorm as many problem-solvers as you can):

_____

_____

_____

From your list, choose the best solutions and develop
strategies for success.

_____

_____

_____

Reflections: Journal how you're feeling, your successes, anything that comes to mind about your progress so far. Read through *The 17 Day Diet* book to learn about all my strategies for overcoming barriers. Which ones can you apply today?

_____

_____

_____

_____

_____

_____

DAY 8—MY DAILY FOOD CHART   DATE

Dr. Mike's Food Tip of the Day

Gauge instead of gorge . . . Just because you *can* eat it doesn't mean you should! Remember to gauge how full you are and stop eating before you are stuffed. If you forget (or choose) to leave off your second dairy or carb serving, that's just fine. Cycle 3 is all about learning to listen to your body so you will eat when you are hungry and eat only until you are full.

WEIGHT

WATER INTAKE

number of 8-ounce glasses

☐ ☐ ☐ ☐
☐ ☐ ☐ ☐

FOOD INTAKE

number of servings

☐ Lean Proteins

☐ Cleansing Vegetables

☐ Natural Starch/ High-Fiber Cereal/or Pasta (2 servings)

☐ Fruit (2 servings)

☐ Probiotic Foods/ Dairy/Dairy Subs (1–2 servings)

☐ Friendly Fats (1–2 tablespoons)

☐ Optional Snack

Breakfast

_____
_____
_____
_____
_____

Lunch

_____
_____
_____
_____

Dinner

_____
_____
_____
_____

Snacks

_____
_____

Dr. Mike's Workout Tip of the Day

Regular cardiovascular exercise is not only helping you lose weight but is improving your overall health in multiple ways. Improvements in blood pressure and cholesterol levels, and prevention of osteoporosis, heart disease, type 2 diabetes, and even some forms of cancer can be attributed to regular physical activity.

Cardio

DATE	ACTIVITY DESCRIPTION	DURATION	CALORIES BURNED	DISTANCE	STEPS

Toning Exercises

EXERCISES	SETS	REPS	WEIGHT	TIME	CALORIES BURNED

DAY 8—MY DAILY JOURNAL

What worked well?

_____
_____
_____

What didn't work well?

_____
_____
_____

I experienced the following challenges:

_____
_____
_____

Ways to overcome these challenges
(brainstorm as many problem-solvers as you can):

_____
_____
_____

From your list, choose the best solutions and develop
strategies for success.

_____
_____
_____

Reflections: Journal how you're feeling, your successes, anything that
comes to mind about your progress so far. Read through *The 17 Day Diet*
book to learn about all my strategies for overcoming barriers. Which
ones can you apply today?

_____
_____
_____
_____
_____
_____
_____

DAY 9—MY DAILY FOOD CHART   DATE

Dr. Mike's Food Tip of the Day

Are you a reformed "mindless eater"? Eating while watching TV or reading can easily cause you to munch mindlessly. That's why learning portion control is so important to lasting weight-loss success. Measure out the amount of food you are allowed, then eat without guilt!

WEIGHT

WATER INTAKE

number of 8-ounce glasses

☐ ☐ ☐ ☐
☐ ☐ ☐ ☐

FOOD INTAKE

number of servings

☐ Lean Proteins

☐ Cleansing Vegetables

☐ Natural Starch/ High-Fiber Cereal/or Pasta (2 servings)

☐ Fruit (2 servings)

☐ Probiotic Foods/ Dairy/Dairy Subs (1–2 servings)

☐ Friendly Fats (1–2 tablespoons)

☐ Optional Snack

Breakfast

Lunch

Dinner

Snacks

Dr. Mike's Workout Tip of the Day

Instead of settling into one activity and not deviating from it, try cross-training, which allows you to use different muscle groups, thus helping to prevent overuse injuries. You will be in better condition overall, as different muscles are worked while others recover. Think of adding a new type of exercise to your routine this week.

Cardio

DATE	ACTIVITY DESCRIPTION	DURATION	CALORIES BURNED	DISTANCE	STEPS

Toning Exercises

EXERCISES	SETS	REPS	WEIGHT	TIME	CALORIES BURNED

DAY 9—MY DAILY JOURNAL

What worked well?

_____
_____
_____

What didn't work well?

_____
_____
_____

I experienced the following challenges:

_____
_____
_____

**Ways to overcome these challenges
(brainstorm as many problem-solvers as you can):**

_____
_____
_____

**From your list, choose the best solutions and develop
strategies for success.**

_____
_____
_____

Reflections: Journal how you're feeling, your successes, anything that
comes to mind about your progress so far. Read through *The 17 Day Diet*
book to learn about all my strategies for overcoming barriers. Which
ones can you apply today?

_____
_____
_____
_____
_____
_____
_____

DAY 10—MY DAILY FOOD CHART   DATE

Dr. Mike's Food Tip of the Day

Are you really hungry or could you be thirsty instead? It's easy to know you are thirsty after a workout or when you've just finished mowing the lawn. Sometimes we get a feeling in our stomach that makes us think we are hungry when our body is actually getting a bit dehydrated. Next time you feel that hunger signal, drink a glass of water first. If after a few minutes you still have that empty feeling, follow those hunger pangs to the kitchen for a healthy snack!

WEIGHT

WATER INTAKE

number of 8-ounce glasses

☐ ☐ ☐ ☐
☐ ☐ ☐ ☐

FOOD INTAKE

number of servings

☐ Lean Proteins

☐ Cleansing
Vegetables

☐ Natural Starch/
High-Fiber
Cereal/or Pasta
(2 servings)

☐ Fruit
(2 servings)

☐ Probiotic Foods/
Dairy/Dairy Subs
(1–2 servings)

☐ Friendly Fats
(1–2 tablespoons)

☐ Optional Snack

Breakfast

_____
_____
_____
_____
_____

Lunch

_____
_____
_____
_____

Dinner

_____
_____
_____
_____

Snacks

_____
_____

Dr. Mike's Workout Tip of the Day

Improved digestion and better bowel habits are two more benefits of regular exercise. Working out improves blood circulation and oxygen flow throughout the body, which helps to keep waste products moving through your digestive system and eliminated without delay. Get moving, and so will your digestive system.

Cardio

DATE	ACTIVITY DESCRIPTION	DURATION	CALORIES BURNED	DISTANCE	STEPS

Toning Exercises

EXERCISES	SETS	REPS	WEIGHT	TIME	CALORIES BURNED

DAY 10—MY DAILY JOURNAL

What worked well?

_____
_____
_____

What didn't work well?

_____
_____
_____

I experienced the following challenges:

_____
_____
_____

Ways to overcome these challenges
(brainstorm as many problem-solvers as you can):

_____
_____
_____

From your list, choose the best solutions and develop
strategies for success.

_____
_____
_____

Reflections: Journal how you're feeling, your successes, anything that
comes to mind about your progress so far. Read through *The 17 Day Diet*
book to learn about all my strategies for overcoming barriers. Which
ones can you apply today?

_____
_____
_____
_____
_____
_____

DAY 11—MY DAILY FOOD CHART   DATE

Dr. Mike's Food Tip of the Day

Get enough sleep so you don't overeat! University of Chicago researchers have concluded that lack of sleep disrupts two hormones that regulate appetite—leptin, a hormone that tells the brain when it is time to eat, and ghrelin, a hormone that triggers hunger. Without enough sleep (8 hours for most of us), you may begin to crave foods high in carbohydrates, calories, fat, and sugar.

WEIGHT

WATER INTAKE

number of 8-ounce glasses

☐ ☐ ☐ ☐
☐ ☐ ☐ ☐

FOOD INTAKE
number of servings

☐ Lean Proteins

☐ Cleansing Vegetables

☐ Natural Starch/ High-Fiber Cereal/or Pasta (2 servings)

☐ Fruit (2 servings)

☐ Probiotic Foods/ Dairy/Dairy Subs (1–2 servings)

☐ Friendly Fats (1–2 tablespoons)

☐ Optional Snack

Breakfast

Lunch

Dinner

Snacks

Dr. Mike's Workout Tip of the Day

Straighten that sedentary slump! Aerobic exercise, strength-training exercises, and stretching exercises work together to improve bad posture. Aerobic exercises help back muscles to become less stiff and more flexible, while strength-training strengthens your back, shoulders, and stomach muscles. Also try Pilates and yoga classes for improvement in posture and flexibility.

Cardio

DATE	ACTIVITY DESCRIPTION	DURATION	CALORIES BURNED	DISTANCE	STEPS

Toning Exercises

EXERCISES	SETS	REPS	WEIGHT	TIME	CALORIES BURNED

DAY 11—MY DAILY JOURNAL

What worked well?

_____
_____
_____

What didn't work well?

_____
_____
_____

I experienced the following challenges:

_____
_____
_____

**Ways to overcome these challenges
(brainstorm as many problem-solvers as you can):**

_____
_____
_____

**From your list, choose the best solutions and develop
strategies for success.**

_____
_____
_____

Reflections: Journal how you're feeling, your successes, anything that
comes to mind about your progress so far. Read through *The 17 Day Diet*
book to learn about all my strategies for overcoming barriers. Which
ones can you apply today?

_____
_____
_____
_____
_____
_____

DAY 12—MY DAILY FOOD CHART   DATE

Dr. Mike's Food Tip of the Day

Need that chocolate fix? If giving up chocolate has been a challenge for you on the 17 Day Diet, now that you are on Cycle 3, chocolate can once again be part of your life! Check out the light chocolate ice cream bars in the freezer case of your supermarket. Skinny Cow, Weight Watchers, and no-sugar-added Fudgsicle frozen bars await!

WEIGHT

WATER INTAKE

number of 8-ounce glasses

☐ ☐ ☐ ☐
☐ ☐ ☐ ☐

FOOD INTAKE

number of servings

☐ Lean Proteins

☐ Cleansing
Vegetables

☐ Natural Starch/
High-Fiber
Cereal/or Pasta
(2 servings)

☐ Fruit
(2 servings)

☐ Probiotic Foods/
Dairy/Dairy Subs
(1–2 servings)

☐ Friendly Fats
(1–2 tablespoons)

☐ Optional Snack

Breakfast

_____
_____
_____
_____
_____

Lunch

_____
_____
_____
_____

Dinner

_____
_____
_____
_____

Snacks

_____
_____

Dr. Mike's Workout Tip of the Day

Have you heard the phrase "Not exercising is not an option"? I hope that you feel this way by now and have made a commitment to daily exercise. While others may feel that exercising four to six days a week is enough to maintain a good fitness level, I recommend setting a daily goal. If you commit to it, you will be less likely to make excuses.

Cardio

DATE	ACTIVITY DESCRIPTION	DURATION	CALORIES BURNED	DISTANCE	STEPS

Toning Exercises

EXERCISES	SETS	REPS	WEIGHT	TIME	CALORIES BURNED

DAY 12—MY DAILY JOURNAL

What worked well?

_____
_____
_____

What didn't work well?

_____
_____
_____

I experienced the following challenges:

_____
_____
_____

Ways to overcome these challenges
(brainstorm as many problem-solvers as you can):

_____
_____
_____

From your list, choose the best solutions and develop
strategies for success.

_____
_____
_____

Reflections: Journal how you're feeling, your successes, anything that
comes to mind about your progress so far. Read through *The 17 Day Diet*
book to learn about all my strategies for overcoming barriers. Which
ones can you apply today?

_____
_____
_____
_____
_____
_____

DAY 13—MY DAILY FOOD CHART   DATE

Dr. Mike's Food Tip of the Day

Have you always been a fast eater? If so, here are a couple of tips to slow down your eating, which will allow your brain to register that you are full: Chew every bite at least 10 times. It'll help your digestion, too! Put down your fork (or spoon) between bites. This will force you to break the "wolf it down" syndrome.

WEIGHT

WATER INTAKE

number of 8-ounce glasses

☐ ☐ ☐ ☐
☐ ☐ ☐ ☐

FOOD INTAKE

number of servings

☐ Lean Proteins

☐ Cleansing Vegetables

☐ Natural Starch/ High-Fiber Cereal/or Pasta (2 servings)

☐ Fruit (2 servings)

☐ Probiotic Foods/ Dairy/Dairy Subs (1–2 servings)

☐ Friendly Fats (1–2 tablespoons)

☐ Optional Snack

Breakfast

_____
_____
_____
_____

Lunch

_____
_____
_____
_____

Dinner

_____
_____
_____
_____

Snacks

_____
_____

Dr. Mike's Workout Tip of the Day

During Cycle 2, I extolled the virtues of using a pedometer. Lots of other fitness gadgets are also on the market that you may find helpful to reaching your fitness goals. Besides the 17 Day Diet's companion exercise DVD, *The 17 Minute Workout* (order at www.the17daydiet .com), there are heart rate monitors, exercise bands, tubes, balls, and a plethora of iPhone and iPod training apps. Happy fitness shopping!

Cardio

DATE	ACTIVITY DESCRIPTION	DURATION	CALORIES BURNED	DISTANCE	STEPS

Toning Exercises

EXERCISES	SETS	REPS	WEIGHT	TIME	CALORIES BURNED

DAY 13—MY DAILY JOURNAL

What worked well?

_____

_____

_____

What didn't work well?

_____

_____

_____

I experienced the following challenges:

_____

_____

_____

Ways to overcome these challenges
(brainstorm as many problem-solvers as you can):

_____

_____

_____

From your list, choose the best solutions and develop
strategies for success.

_____

_____

_____

Reflections: Journal how you're feeling, your successes, anything that
comes to mind about your progress so far. Read through *The 17 Day Diet*
book to learn about all my strategies for overcoming barriers. Which
ones can you apply today?

_____

_____

_____

_____

_____

_____

_____

DAY 14—MY DAILY FOOD CHART   DATE

Dr. Mike's Food Tip of the Day

Here are a couple more tips to break the "gulp and go" habit: Try using chopsticks instead of a fork and spoon to eat your next meal. Between bites, take a small sip of water. Eat with others whenever possible. Make a conscious effort to participate in the conversation, which will naturally slow down your eating.

WEIGHT

WATER INTAKE

number of 8-ounce glasses

☐ ☐ ☐ ☐
☐ ☐ ☐ ☐

FOOD INTAKE

number of servings

☐ Lean Proteins

☐ Cleansing
Vegetables

☐ Natural Starch/
High-Fiber
Cereal/or Pasta
(2 servings)

☐ Fruit
(2 servings)

☐ Probiotic Foods/
Dairy/Dairy Subs
(1–2 servings)

☐ Friendly Fats
(1–2 tablespoons)

☐ Optional Snack

Breakfast

_____

_____

_____

_____

_____

Lunch

_____

_____

_____

_____

_____

Dinner

_____

_____

_____

_____

Snacks

_____

_____

_____

Dr. Mike's Workout Tip of the Day

Exercising with your pet can be beneficial for both of you! Dogs need exercise, too; in fact, it's been reported that 25–40 percent of them are overweight or obese. It's always more fun to exercise with a companion, so if you haven't already, try including your pooch next time you think of heading out for a hike.

Cardio

DATE	ACTIVITY DESCRIPTION	DURATION	CALORIES BURNED	DISTANCE	STEPS

Toning Exercises

EXERCISES	SETS	REPS	WEIGHT	TIME	CALORIES BURNED

DAY 14—MY DAILY JOURNAL

What worked well?

_____

_____

_____

What didn't work well?

_____

_____

_____

I experienced the following challenges:

_____

_____

_____

Ways to overcome these challenges
(brainstorm as many problem-solvers as you can):

_____

_____

_____

From your list, choose the best solutions and develop
strategies for success.

_____

_____

_____

Reflections: Journal how you're feeling, your successes, anything that
comes to mind about your progress so far. Read through *The 17 Day Diet*
book to learn about all my strategies for overcoming barriers. Which
ones can you apply today?

_____

_____

_____

_____

_____

_____

DAY 15—MY DAILY FOOD CHART   DATE

Dr. Mike's Food Tip of the Day

Take the focus off food. Make meals more about spending quality time with family and friends and you'll soon find mealtimes, both the regular, everyday ones and the special occasions, will revolve less around food and more about the memories you are making around the dinner table.

WEIGHT

WATER INTAKE

number of 8-ounce glasses

☐ ☐ ☐ ☐
☐ ☐ ☐ ☐

FOOD INTAKE

number of servings

☐ Lean Proteins

☐ Cleansing
Vegetables

☐ Natural Starch/
High-Fiber
Cereal/or Pasta
(2 servings)

☐ Fruit
(2 servings)

☐ Probiotic Foods/
Dairy/Dairy Subs
(1–2 servings)

☐ Friendly Fats
(1–2 tablespoons)

☐ Optional Snack

Breakfast

_____

_____

_____

_____

_____

Lunch

_____

_____

_____

_____

Dinner

_____

_____

_____

_____

Snacks

_____

_____

Dr. Mike's Workout Tip of the Day

You have almost completed Cycle 3, so let's talk about setbacks. The best way to deal with a setback in your food or fitness goals is first to acknowledge it, then think about why it happened and what you can do to prevent it from happening again. Try not to beat yourself up for blowing off your workout or eating that dessert, and make a fresh start tomorrow.

Cardio

DATE	ACTIVITY DESCRIPTION	DURATION	CALORIES BURNED	DISTANCE	STEPS

Toning Exercises

EXERCISES	SETS	REPS	WEIGHT	TIME	CALORIES BURNED

DAY 15—MY DAILY JOURNAL

What worked well?

_____

_____

_____

What didn't work well?

_____

_____

_____

I experienced the following challenges:

_____

_____

_____

Ways to overcome these challenges
(brainstorm as many problem-solvers as you can):

_____

_____

_____

From your list, choose the best solutions and develop
strategies for success.

_____

_____

_____

Reflections: Journal how you're feeling, your successes, anything that
comes to mind about your progress so far. Read through *The 17 Day Diet*
book to learn about all my strategies for overcoming barriers. Which
ones can you apply today?

_____

_____

_____

_____

_____

_____

DAY 16—MY DAILY FOOD CHART   DATE

Dr. Mike's Food Tip of the Day

Did you used to be a meal skipper? Maybe you often skipped meals because you thought it would help you lose weight, or you thought you were too busy to eat. Hopefully, by now you realize it's better to eat at regular intervals throughout the day to keep your metabolism elevated so your body doesn't go into starvation mode. If you used to skip meals, don't allow yourself to slip back into that harmful habit.

WEIGHT

WATER INTAKE

number of 8-ounce glasses

☐ ☐ ☐ ☐
☐ ☐ ☐ ☐

FOOD INTAKE

number of servings

☐ Lean Proteins

☐ Cleansing
  Vegetables

☐ Natural Starch/
  High-Fiber
  Cereal/or Pasta
  (2 servings)

☐ Fruit
  (2 servings)

☐ Probiotic Foods/
  Dairy/Dairy Subs
  (1–2 servings)

☐ Friendly Fats
  (1–2 tablespoons)

☐ Optional Snack

Breakfast

_____
_____
_____
_____
_____

Lunch

_____
_____
_____
_____

Dinner

_____
_____
_____
_____

Snacks

_____
_____
_____

Dr. Mike's Workout Tip of the Day

Get fit, not flabby! While weight loss can be accomplished without exercise, those who fail to move their bodies lose weight and muscle tone at the same time. Toning muscles as weight is lost helps eliminate excess flab.

Cardio

DATE	ACTIVITY DESCRIPTION	DURATION	CALORIES BURNED	DISTANCE	STEPS

Toning Exercises

EXERCISES	SETS	REPS	WEIGHT	TIME	CALORIES BURNED

DAY 16—MY DAILY JOURNAL

What worked well?

_____

_____

_____

What didn't work well?

_____

_____

_____

I experienced the following challenges:

_____

_____

_____

Ways to overcome these challenges
(brainstorm as many problem-solvers as you can):

_____

_____

_____

From your list, choose the best solutions and develop
strategies for success.

_____

_____

_____

Reflections: Journal how you're feeling, your successes, anything that
comes to mind about your progress so far. Read through *The 17 Day Diet*
book to learn about all my strategies for overcoming barriers. Which
ones can you apply today?

_____

_____

_____

_____

_____

_____

DAY 17—MY DAILY FOOD CHART   DATE

Dr. Mike's Food Tip of the Day

A food-mood connection has been made involving serotonin, a neu-
rotransmitter in the brain that can affect everything from mood to
metabolism and sleep to sexuality. The food connection is made
because serotonin is made from tryptophan, found in lots of foods:
turkey, red meat, fish and shellfish, beans, oats, nuts, and seeds, to
name some of them. When tryptophan's consumed with carbs, in
particular, serotonin levels rise and mood improves, too!

WEIGHT

WATER INTAKE

number of 8-ounce glasses

☐ ☐ ☐ ☐
☐ ☐ ☐ ☐

FOOD INTAKE

number of servings

☐ Lean Proteins

☐ Cleansing
Vegetables

☐ Natural Starch/
High-Fiber
Cereal/or Pasta
(2 servings)

☐ Fruit
(2 servings)

☐ Probiotic Foods/
Dairy/Dairy Subs
(1–2 servings)

☐ Friendly Fats
(1–2 tablespoons)

☐ Optional Snack

Breakfast

Lunch

Dinner

Snacks

Dr. Mike's Workout Tip of the Day

Exercising with a cold can actually help speed up your recovery, so don't let a run-of-the-mill rhinovirus stop you from going for a 30- to 45-minute walk. Just leave your intense workout for another day. If you have flu symptoms, however—fever, aches, chest congestion, swollen glands—exercising can make things worse. After your fever is gone and you are symptom-free, you can begin to exercise moderately.

Cardio

DATE	ACTIVITY DESCRIPTION	DURATION	CALORIES BURNED	DISTANCE	STEPS

Toning Exercises

EXERCISES	SETS	REPS	WEIGHT	TIME	CALORIES BURNED

DAY 17—MY DAILY JOURNAL

What worked well?

_____

_____

_____

What didn't work well?

_____

_____

_____

I experienced the following challenges:

_____

_____

_____

**Ways to overcome these challenges
(brainstorm as many problem-solvers as you can):**

_____

_____

_____

**From your list, choose the best solutions and develop
strategies for success.**

_____

_____

_____

Reflections: Journal how you're feeling, your successes, anything that comes to mind about your progress so far. Read through *The 17 Day Diet* book to learn about all my strategies for overcoming barriers. Which ones can you apply today?

_____

_____

_____

_____

_____

_____

Review: Weight-Loss Checklist—Cycle 3

* *

You've been following the 17 Day Diet for more than a month now. Are you finding any of these obstacles standing in the way of your weight loss?

1. Am I liable to overeat at certain times of day or on certain days of the week?

    ☐ **Always**   ☐ **Sometimes**   ☐ **Rarely or Never**

2. Are my portion sizes larger than they should be?

    ☐ **Always**   ☐ **Sometimes**   ☐ **Rarely or Never**

3. Am I eating while driving?

    ☐ **Always**   ☐ **Sometimes**   ☐ **Rarely or Never**

4. Am I eating at times I shouldn't, when I'm bored or stressed?

    ☐ **Always**   ☐ **Sometimes**   ☐ **Rarely or Never**

5. Am I making excuses for not working out on a daily basis?

    ☐ **Always**   ☐ **Sometimes**   ☐ **Rarely or Never**

My top areas to work on in the next cycle:

_____

_____

_____

_____

I lost _____ pounds on Cycle 3.

What positive new lifestyle patterns and habits are emerging in your life now? List as many as you can think of.

_____

_____

_____

_____

_____

_____

_____

_____

_____

_____

_____

_____

_____

_____

_____

_____

_____

_____

_____

_____

_____

_____

_____

_____

_____

_____

_____

_____

I have met/have not yet met my goal. Circle the one that applies.

If you have not met your goal, let's talk about what to do next. You have several choices:

- Begin with Cycle 1 and work your way back through the cycles.
- If you're very close to your goal, stay on Cycle 1 until you reach it.
- Use Cycle 2, then 3, to reach your goal.
- Stay on Cycle 3 until you reach your goal.

  Which strategy will you use?

CYCLE 4

. . . .

Arrive

GOAL

To keep you at your goal weight through a program of eating that lets you enjoy your favorite foods on weekends, while eating healthfully during the week.

Start the Arrive Cycle

The Arrive Cycle is unique in that it helps you keep your weight off, while letting you enjoy yourself and eat freely from your favorite foods on weekends.

Basically, the Arrive Cycle works like this:

- Monday breakfast through Friday lunch: Enjoy meal plans from one of your favorite cycles (Accelerate, Activate, or Achieve).

- Friday dinner through Sunday dinner: Enjoy your favorite foods and meals in moderation over the weekend.

- Enjoy no more than 1 to 3 favorite meals over the weekend. Do not binge. Eat slowly and enjoy your food.

- If you desire, enjoy alcoholic drinks in moderation over the weekend (1 to 2 daily): 1½ ounces hard liquor or 5 ounces wine or 12 ounces beer.

- You may include soups in your daily menus, as long as they are broth based. Avoid soups made with milk or cream. Having soup prior to a meal will help curb your appetite and help you feel full.

- As one of your fruit servings, you may substitute fruit juice (unsweetened), but no more than ¾ cup per serving.

- Feel free to enjoy 1 cup of vegetable juice as a snack.

- Continue to use condiments in moderation. Choose nonfat, low-calorie seasonings, such as reduced-fat dressings, spices, herbs, lemon or lime juice, vinegar, and hot sauce.

- Exercise on weekends, as well as weekdays.

- Each Monday, I'd like you to renew your commitment to yourself and to your new incredible body. Do this and you'll control your eating week by week with a strategy that'll guarantee success.

DAY 1—MY DAILY FOOD CHART   DATE

Dr. Mike's Food Tip of the Day

What foods have you missed? Enchiladas and chips with queso dip?
Kung pao chicken and egg rolls? Fettuccine Alfredo and tiramisu? Now
that you have arrived at your goal weight (applause, applause!), strate-
gic cheating on the weekends is your reward. Enjoy up to three of your
favorite meals over the weekend. Splurge a little but don't binge!

WEIGHT

WATER INTAKE

number of 8-ounce glasses

☐ ☐ ☐ ☐
☐ ☐ ☐ ☐

FOOD INTAKE

number of servings

☐ Lean Proteins

☐ Cleansing
Vegetables

☐ Natural Starch/
High-Fiber
Cereal/or Pasta
(2 servings)

☐ Fruit
(2 servings)

☐ Probiotic Foods/
Dairy/Dairy Subs
(1–2 servings)

☐ Friendly Fats
(1–2 tablespoons)

☐ Optional Snack

Breakfast

Lunch

Dinner

Snacks

Dr. Mike's Workout Tip of the Day

Medically speaking, reaching your goal weight is one of the best things you have done for your health. And it's thanks, in large part, to leading a more active life. Make sure to schedule a checkup with your doctor to monitor your blood pressure, cholesterol, and blood sugar since you have completed the first three cycles of the 17 Day Diet.

Cardio

DATE	ACTIVITY DESCRIPTION	DURATION	CALORIES BURNED	DISTANCE	STEPS

Toning Exercises

EXERCISES	SETS	REPS	WEIGHT	TIME	CALORIES BURNED

DAY 1—MY DAILY JOURNAL

What worked well?

_____

_____

_____

What didn't work well?

_____

_____

_____

I experienced the following challenges:

_____

_____

_____

Ways to overcome these challenges
(brainstorm as many problem-solvers as you can):

_____

_____

_____

From your list, choose the best solutions and develop
strategies for success.

_____

_____

_____

Reflections: Journal how you're feeling, your successes, anything that
comes to mind about your progress so far. Read through *The 17 Day Diet*
book to learn about all my strategies for overcoming barriers. Which
ones can you apply today?

_____

_____

_____

_____

_____

_____

DAY 2—MY DAILY FOOD CHART   DATE

Dr. Mike's Food Tip of the Day

To stay in control of portions when dining out, ask for half of your entrée to be boxed up before it appears on your plate. Fill up on salad, sans the croutons and cheese. Light dressing on the side, please!

WEIGHT

WATER INTAKE

number of 8-ounce glasses

☐ ☐ ☐ ☐
☐ ☐ ☐ ☐

FOOD INTAKE

number of servings

☐ Lean Proteins

☐ Cleansing Vegetables

☐ Natural Starch/ High-Fiber Cereal/or Pasta (2 servings)

☐ Fruit (2 servings)

☐ Probiotic Foods/ Dairy/Dairy Subs (1–2 servings)

☐ Friendly Fats (1–2 tablespoons)

☐ Optional Snack

Breakfast

_____
_____
_____
_____
_____

Lunch

_____
_____
_____
_____
_____

Dinner

_____
_____
_____
_____

Snacks

_____
_____
_____

Dr. Mike's Workout Tip of the Day

No wonder our ancestors who farmed the land could eat anything they wanted and not gain weight! Farming, baling hay, and other chores can burn between 500 and 600 calories per hour! Maybe you're not going to drive to the country and help clean out a barn, but how about tackling that overloaded garage this weekend?

Cardio

DATE	ACTIVITY DESCRIPTION	DURATION	CALORIES BURNED	DISTANCE	STEPS

Toning Exercises

EXERCISES	SETS	REPS	WEIGHT	TIME	CALORIES BURNED

DAY 2—MY DAILY JOURNAL

What worked well?

_____
_____
_____

What didn't work well?

_____
_____
_____

I experienced the following challenges:

_____
_____
_____

Ways to overcome these challenges
(brainstorm as many problem-solvers as you can):

_____
_____
_____

From your list, choose the best solutions and develop
strategies for success.

_____
_____
_____

Reflections: Journal how you're feeling, your successes, anything that
comes to mind about your progress so far. Read through *The 17 Day Diet*
book to learn about all my strategies for overcoming barriers. Which
ones can you apply today?

_____
_____
_____
_____
_____
_____

DAY 3—MY DAILY FOOD CHART   DATE

Dr. Mike's Food Tip of the Day

Keeping weight off after you've lost it is made easier when you make healthier substitutes all or most of the time. You use mustard instead of mayo on sandwiches, you purchase skim instead of 2 percent or whole milk, and you choose fat-free, sugar-free ice cream and frozen treats. Make it a mind-set—a part of your lifestyle, not a diet.

WEIGHT

WATER INTAKE
number of 8-ounce glasses

☐ ☐ ☐ ☐
☐ ☐ ☐ ☐

FOOD INTAKE
number of servings

☐ Lean Proteins

☐ Cleansing Vegetables

☐ Natural Starch/ High-Fiber Cereal/or Pasta (2 servings)

☐ Fruit (2 servings)

☐ Probiotic Foods/ Dairy/Dairy Subs (1–2 servings)

☐ Friendly Fats (1–2 tablespoons)

☐ Optional Snack

Breakfast

Lunch

Dinner

Snacks

Dr. Mike's Workout Tip of the Day

Have you thought about setting a fitness challenge for yourself, now that you are down to your goal weight? Think about signing up for the next charity walk or run in your community. You'll be helping out a worthy cause while helping your fine, fit self stay that way!

Cardio

DATE	ACTIVITY DESCRIPTION	DURATION	CALORIES BURNED	DISTANCE	STEPS

Toning Exercises

EXERCISES	SETS	REPS	WEIGHT	TIME	CALORIES BURNED

DAY 3—MY DAILY JOURNAL

What worked well?

_____

_____

_____

What didn't work well?

_____

_____

_____

I experienced the following challenges:

_____

_____

_____

Ways to overcome these challenges
(brainstorm as many problem-solvers as you can):

_____

_____

_____

From your list, choose the best solutions and develop
strategies for success.

_____

_____

_____

Reflections: Journal how you're feeling, your successes, anything that
comes to mind about your progress so far. Read through *The 17 Day Diet*
book to learn about all my strategies for overcoming barriers. Which
ones can you apply today?

_____

_____

_____

_____

_____

_____

_____

DAY 4—MY DAILY FOOD CHART   DATE

Dr. Mike's Food Tip of the Day

Careful! Don't pull the trigger . . . on the foods that spell trouble for you. Are potato chips a trouble food for you? Is it hard to eat 15 chips and stop? How about chocolate? Can you eat three Hershey's Kisses and go on your way? If there are certain foods that can cause you to go into binge mode, you may have to eliminate them from your life, not just from your weekend treat meals.

WEIGHT

WATER INTAKE

number of 8-ounce glasses

☐ ☐ ☐ ☐
☐ ☐ ☐ ☐

FOOD INTAKE

number of servings

☐ Lean Proteins

☐ Cleansing
   Vegetables

☐ Natural Starch/
   High-Fiber
   Cereal/or Pasta
   (2 servings)

☐ Fruit
   (2 servings)

☐ Probiotic Foods/
   Dairy/Dairy Subs
   (1–2 servings)

☐ Friendly Fats
   (1–2 tablespoons)

☐ Optional Snack

Breakfast

_____
_____
_____
_____
_____

Lunch

_____
_____
_____
_____

Dinner

_____
_____
_____

Snacks

_____
_____

Dr. Mike's Workout Tip of the Day

Should you let the housekeeper go? Clean your own house and you'll burn about 250 calories per hour and put extra dollars in your budget for—what else? A new pair of workout shoes!

Cardio

DATE	ACTIVITY DESCRIPTION	DURATION	CALORIES BURNED	DISTANCE	STEPS

Toning Exercises

EXERCISES	SETS	REPS	WEIGHT	TIME	CALORIES BURNED

DAY 4—MY DAILY JOURNAL

What worked well?

_____

_____

_____

What didn't work well?

_____

_____

_____

I experienced the following challenges:

_____

_____

_____

Ways to overcome these challenges
(brainstorm as many problem-solvers as you can):

_____

_____

_____

From your list, choose the best solutions and develop
strategies for success.

_____

_____

_____

Reflections: Journal how you're feeling, your successes, anything that
comes to mind about your progress so far. Read through *The 17 Day Diet*
book to learn about all my strategies for overcoming barriers. Which
ones can you apply today?

_____

_____

_____

_____

_____

_____

_____

DAY 5—MY DAILY FOOD CHART   DATE

Dr. Mike's Food Tip of the Day

Love your body. Change the way you dress to flatter your physique. Some clothes make you look much heavier than you are. Look for fabrics and styles that make you look thinner before you lose even a pound of fat. Change your hairstyle and, if necessary, color it. Take care of your skin. Looking better can help you follow the program more effectively.

WEIGHT

WATER INTAKE

number of 8-ounce glasses

☐ ☐ ☐ ☐
☐ ☐ ☐ ☐

FOOD INTAKE

number of servings

☐ Lean Proteins

☐ Cleansing Vegetables

☐ Natural Starch/ High-Fiber Cereal/or Pasta (2 servings)

☐ Fruit (2 servings)

☐ Probiotic Foods/ Dairy/Dairy Subs (1–2 servings)

☐ Friendly Fats (1–2 tablespoons)

☐ Optional Snack

Breakfast

_____
_____
_____
_____
_____

Lunch

_____
_____
_____
_____

Dinner

_____
_____
_____
_____

Snacks

_____
_____

Dr. Mike's Workout Tip of the Day

What is your "new normal"? Just think for a moment about how you were spending your leisure hours before the 17 Day Diet, and what has become your new normal . . . Do you recognize the couch potato who rarely walked for the sake of walking to improve fitness levels, as well as health? Change *can* come quickly, if you are committed to it.

Cardio

DATE	ACTIVITY DESCRIPTION	DURATION	CALORIES BURNED	DISTANCE	STEPS

Toning Exercises

EXERCISES	SETS	REPS	WEIGHT	TIME	CALORIES BURNED

DAY 5—MY DAILY JOURNAL

What worked well?

_____

_____

_____

What didn't work well?

_____

_____

_____

I experienced the following challenges:

_____

_____

_____

Ways to overcome these challenges
(brainstorm as many problem-solvers as you can):

_____

_____

_____

From your list, choose the best solutions and develop
strategies for success.

_____

_____

_____

Reflections: Journal how you're feeling, your successes, anything that
comes to mind about your progress so far. Read through *The 17 Day Diet*
book to learn about all my strategies for overcoming barriers. Which
ones can you apply today?

_____

_____

_____

_____

_____

_____

DAY 6—MY DAILY FOOD CHART   DATE

Dr. Mike's Food Tip of the Day

"If you always do what you always did, you'll always get what you always got." Keep this mantra front and center on your refrigerator, along with a photo of your fine-lookin' new self! You have changed the way you think about food and have seen results. You have formed new habits and have committed to a different lifestyle in less than two months. Celebrate your success!

WEIGHT

WATER INTAKE

number of 8-ounce glasses

☐ ☐ ☐ ☐
☐ ☐ ☐ ☐

FOOD INTAKE

number of servings

☐ Lean Proteins

☐ Cleansing Vegetables

☐ Natural Starch/ High-Fiber Cereal/or Pasta (2 servings)

☐ Fruit (2 servings)

☐ Probiotic Foods/ Dairy/Dairy Subs (1–2 servings)

☐ Friendly Fats (1–2 tablespoons)

☐ Optional Snack

Breakfast

Lunch

Dinner

Snacks

Dr. Mike's Workout Tip of the Day

Lifestyle activities are easy to incorporate into your daily routine over the long haul. That doesn't mean you will be abandoning your workouts. You will just be burning more calories automatically!

Cardio

DATE	ACTIVITY DESCRIPTION	DURATION	CALORIES BURNED	DISTANCE	STEPS

Toning Exercises

EXERCISES	SETS	REPS	WEIGHT	TIME	CALORIES BURNED

DAY 6—MY DAILY JOURNAL

What worked well?

_____
_____
_____

What didn't work well?

_____
_____
_____

I experienced the following challenges:

_____
_____
_____

Ways to overcome these challenges
(brainstorm as many problem-solvers as you can):

_____
_____
_____

From your list, choose the best solutions and develop
strategies for success.

_____
_____
_____

Reflections: Journal how you're feeling, your successes, anything that
comes to mind about your progress so far. Read through *The 17 Day Diet*
book to learn about all my strategies for overcoming barriers. Which
ones can you apply today?

_____
_____
_____
_____
_____
_____

DAY 7—MY DAILY FOOD CHART　　　　DATE

Dr. Mike's Food Tip of the Day

It's been a time of discovery. Hopefully, during Cycles 1, 2, and 3, you were exposed to some new foods and preparation methods that you will continue to enjoy for the rest of your life. The deep fryer was in your last garage sale (right?) and has been replaced by low-fat, healthy ways of cooking that leave you satisfied and svelte!

WEIGHT

WATER INTAKE

number of 8-ounce glasses

☐ ☐ ☐ ☐
☐ ☐ ☐ ☐

FOOD INTAKE

number of servings

☐ Lean Proteins

☐ Cleansing Vegetables

☐ Natural Starch/ High-Fiber Cereal/or Pasta (2 servings)

☐ Fruit (2 servings)

☐ Probiotic Foods/ Dairy/Dairy Subs (1–2 servings)

☐ Friendly Fats (1–2 tablespoons)

☐ Optional Snack

Breakfast

Lunch

Dinner

Snacks

Dr. Mike's Workout Tip of the Day

You've heard these before, but now that you are thinner and healthier, maybe you'll take them to heart: Park farther away from your destination and walk. Take the stairs instead of the elevator. When weather permits, take a walk after lunch or during your work break. Walk or ride your bike to the neighborhood market or other locations within a mile or two of your home. Lead a fit life!

Cardio

DATE	ACTIVITY DESCRIPTION	DURATION	CALORIES BURNED	DISTANCE	STEPS

Toning Exercises

EXERCISES	SETS	REPS	WEIGHT	TIME	CALORIES BURNED

DAY 7—MY DAILY JOURNAL

What worked well?

_____
_____
_____

What didn't work well?

_____
_____
_____

I experienced the following challenges:

_____
_____
_____

Ways to overcome these challenges
(brainstorm as many problem-solvers as you can):

_____
_____
_____

From your list, choose the best solutions and develop
strategies for success.

_____
_____
_____

Reflections: Journal how you're feeling, your successes, anything that
comes to mind about your progress so far. Read through *The 17 Day Diet*
book to learn about all my strategies for overcoming barriers. Which
ones can you apply today?

_____
_____
_____
_____
_____
_____
_____

DAY 8—MY DAILY FOOD CHART   DATE

Dr. Mike's Food Tip of the Day

What are you doing to be among the small percentage of dieters who keep their weight off for the long term? The National Weight Control Registry, which has tracked the progress of more than 5,000 dieters since 1994, reports that those who successfully maintain their weight loss continue to eat a low-fat diet, don't skip breakfast, weigh themselves regularly, and exercise daily.

WEIGHT

Breakfast

WATER INTAKE

number of 8-ounce glasses

☐ ☐ ☐ ☐
☐ ☐ ☐ ☐

FOOD INTAKE

number of servings

Lunch

☐ Lean Proteins

☐ Cleansing
Vegetables

☐ Natural Starch/
High-Fiber
Cereal/or Pasta
(2 servings)

Dinner

☐ Fruit
(2 servings)

☐ Probiotic Foods/
Dairy/Dairy Subs
(1–2 servings)

☐ Friendly Fats
(1–2 tablespoons)

Snacks

☐ Optional Snack

Dr. Mike's Workout Tip of the Day

Weekend chores like lawn mowing, which burns nearly 400 calories per hour, and other yard work can help you burn those extra calories you will be consuming on your weekend "free" days. Even getting out and watering the lawn and garden by hand burns just over 100 calories per hour, so get out and stay active!

Cardio

DATE	ACTIVITY DESCRIPTION	DURATION	CALORIES BURNED	DISTANCE	STEPS

Toning Exercises

EXERCISES	SETS	REPS	WEIGHT	TIME	CALORIES BURNED

DAY 8—MY DAILY JOURNAL

What worked well?

_____
_____
_____

What didn't work well?

_____
_____
_____

I experienced the following challenges:

_____
_____
_____

Ways to overcome these challenges
(brainstorm as many problem-solvers as you can):

_____
_____
_____

From your list, choose the best solutions and develop
strategies for success.

_____
_____
_____

Reflections: Journal how you're feeling, your successes, anything that
comes to mind about your progress so far. Read through *The 17 Day Diet*
book to learn about all my strategies for overcoming barriers. Which
ones can you apply today?

_____
_____
_____
_____
_____
_____

DAY 9—MY DAILY FOOD CHART   DATE

Dr. Mike's Food Tip of the Day

"Special orders don't upset us . . ." If you were around in the seventies, you might remember that familiar Burger King commercial that promised they would gladly "Hold the pickle, hold the lettuce . . ." to keep their customers happy! The same thing applies today when you order a restaurant meal. Don't hesitate to ask your server if you can request a particular dish be broiled or baked instead of fried, or if steamed veggies can be substituted for fries.

WEIGHT

WATER INTAKE

number of 8-ounce glasses

☐ ☐ ☐ ☐
☐ ☐ ☐ ☐

FOOD INTAKE

number of servings

☐ Lean Proteins

☐ Cleansing
  Vegetables

☐ Natural Starch/
  High-Fiber
  Cereal/or Pasta
  (2 servings)

☐ Fruit
  (2 servings)

☐ Probiotic Foods/
  Dairy/Dairy Subs
  (1–2 servings)

☐ Friendly Fats
  (1–2 tablespoons)

☐ Optional Snack

Breakfast

_____
_____
_____
_____
_____

Lunch

_____
_____
_____
_____

Dinner

_____
_____
_____
_____

Snacks

_____
_____

Dr. Mike's Workout Tip of the Day

Share and share alike. Have you found a fitness pal in your spouse, significant other, or friend? If you haven't yet persuaded one or more of your nearest and dearest to join you in your daily workout, keep trying. Plan an outing that involves being active, like taking a nature hike. Appeal to their interests, appeal to their health, and appeal to their hearts!

Cardio

DATE	ACTIVITY DESCRIPTION	DURATION	CALORIES BURNED	DISTANCE	STEPS

Toning Exercises

EXERCISES	SETS	REPS	WEIGHT	TIME	CALORIES BURNED

DAY 9—MY DAILY JOURNAL

What worked well?

_____
_____
_____

What didn't work well?

_____
_____
_____

I experienced the following challenges:

_____
_____
_____

**Ways to overcome these challenges
(brainstorm as many problem-solvers as you can):**

_____
_____
_____

**From your list, choose the best solutions and develop
strategies for success.**

_____
_____
_____

Reflections: Journal how you're feeling, your successes, anything that
comes to mind about your progress so far. Read through *The 17 Day Diet*
book to learn about all my strategies for overcoming barriers. Which
ones can you apply today?

_____
_____
_____
_____
_____
_____

DAY 10—MY DAILY FOOD CHART   DATE

Dr. Mike's Food Tip of the Day

The Arrive Cycle cannot be approached as if you've reached the finish line and the race is over. You're still controlling your eating during the week, so you can splurge a bit on the weekends, speeding up your metabolism with the increased calorie intake. If you have a special occasion on a weekday and have that birthday cake and ice cream, enjoy it, but when the weekend rolls around, remember that you've already had your special dessert!

WEIGHT

WATER INTAKE

number of 8-ounce glasses

☐ ☐ ☐ ☐
☐ ☐ ☐ ☐

FOOD INTAKE

number of servings

☐ Lean Proteins

☐ Cleansing Vegetables

☐ Natural Starch/ High-Fiber Cereal/or Pasta (2 servings)

☐ Fruit (2 servings)

☐ Probiotic Foods/ Dairy/Dairy Subs (1–2 servings)

☐ Friendly Fats (1–2 tablespoons)

☐ Optional Snack

Breakfast

_____
_____
_____
_____
_____

Lunch

_____
_____
_____
_____

Dinner

_____
_____
_____
_____

Snacks

_____
_____

Dr. Mike's Workout Tip of the Day

If airports have become your home away from home due to lots of business travel, make sure you travel light with a wheeled bag so you can make use of the time you have before flights to walk the concourse. Wear your pedometer so you can keep track of your steps.

Cardio

DATE	ACTIVITY DESCRIPTION	DURATION	CALORIES BURNED	DISTANCE	STEPS

Toning Exercises

EXERCISES	SETS	REPS	WEIGHT	TIME	CALORIES BURNED

DAY 10—MY DAILY JOURNAL

What worked well?

_____

_____

_____

What didn't work well?

_____

_____

_____

I experienced the following challenges:

_____

_____

_____

**Ways to overcome these challenges
(brainstorm as many problem-solvers as you can):**

_____

_____

_____

**From your list, choose the best solutions and develop
strategies for success.**

_____

_____

_____

Reflections: Journal how you're feeling, your successes, anything that
comes to mind about your progress so far. Read through *The 17 Day Diet*
book to learn about all my strategies for overcoming barriers. Which
ones can you apply today?

_____

_____

_____

_____

_____

_____

DAY 11—MY DAILY FOOD CHART   DATE

Dr. Mike's Food Tip of the Day

Salads, fresh fruit, yogurt, turkey sandwiches, and other healthy foods are readily available in airports these days, so it's up to you to seek them out. Even better, pack a brown bag lunch of your own, including healthy snacks, to eat on the plane or while waiting for your flight.

WEIGHT

WATER INTAKE

number of 8-ounce glasses

☐ ☐ ☐ ☐
☐ ☐ ☐ ☐

FOOD INTAKE

number of servings

☐ Lean Proteins

☐ Cleansing Vegetables

☐ Natural Starch/ High-Fiber Cereal/or Pasta (2 servings)

☐ Fruit (2 servings)

☐ Probiotic Foods/ Dairy/Dairy Subs (1–2 servings)

☐ Friendly Fats (1–2 tablespoons)

☐ Optional Snack

Breakfast

_____

Lunch

_____

Dinner

_____

Snacks

_____

Dr. Mike's Workout Tip of the Day

Think of ways you can make this year's vacation a more active one for you and your family. If your beach holiday has traditionally been spent under an umbrella with a stack of summer reads, read one less book so you can fit in long walks or jogs on the beach. Do some research to plan outings that will involve active exploration wherever you decide to vacation.

Cardio

DATE	ACTIVITY DESCRIPTION	DURATION	CALORIES BURNED	DISTANCE	STEPS

Toning Exercises

EXERCISES	SETS	REPS	WEIGHT	TIME	CALORIES BURNED

DAY 11—MY DAILY JOURNAL

What worked well?

_____

_____

_____

What didn't work well?

_____

_____

_____

I experienced the following challenges:

_____

_____

_____

Ways to overcome these challenges
(brainstorm as many problem-solvers as you can):

_____

_____

_____

From your list, choose the best solutions and develop
strategies for success.

_____

_____

_____

Reflections: Journal how you're feeling, your successes, anything that
comes to mind about your progress so far. Read through *The 17 Day Diet*
book to learn about all my strategies for overcoming barriers. Which
ones can you apply today?

_____

_____

_____

_____

_____

_____

_____

DAY 12—MY DAILY FOOD CHART   DATE

Dr. Mike's Food Tip of the Day

Cooking at home is the best way of staying on track with your eating plan, because you are in total control of the ingredients and methods used to prepare the meal. The calories you burn while cooking are an added benefit—up to 150 an hour!

WEIGHT

WATER INTAKE

number of 8-ounce glasses

☐ ☐ ☐ ☐
☐ ☐ ☐ ☐

FOOD INTAKE

number of servings

☐ Lean Proteins

☐ Cleansing
  Vegetables

☐ Natural Starch/
  High-Fiber
  Cereal/or Pasta
  (2 servings)

☐ Fruit
  (2 servings)

☐ Probiotic Foods/
  Dairy/Dairy Subs
  (1–2 servings)

☐ Friendly Fats
  (1–2 tablespoons)

☐ Optional Snack

Breakfast

_____

_____

_____

_____

_____

Lunch

_____

_____

_____

_____

Dinner

_____

_____

_____

_____

Snacks

_____

_____

_____

Dr. Mike's Workout Tip of the Day

Workout facilities in hotels are the norm these days, so pack your shoes and workout clothes when you travel. Other options are getting out of the hotel for a brisk walk or jog, or using your hotel room as your private gym. Find an exercise class on TV, bring your *17 Minute Workout* DVD (www.the17daydiet.com), or do floor exercises (sit-ups, push-ups, squats, etc.). Oh, and take the stairs instead of the elevator!

Cardio

DATE	ACTIVITY DESCRIPTION	DURATION	CALORIES BURNED	DISTANCE	STEPS

Toning Exercises

EXERCISES	SETS	REPS	WEIGHT	TIME	CALORIES BURNED

DAY 12—MY DAILY JOURNAL

What worked well?

_____

_____

_____

What didn't work well?

_____

_____

_____

I experienced the following challenges:

_____

_____

_____

Ways to overcome these challenges
(brainstorm as many problem-solvers as you can):

_____

_____

_____

From your list, choose the best solutions and develop
strategies for success.

_____

_____

_____

Reflections: Journal how you're feeling, your successes, anything that
comes to mind about your progress so far. Read through *The 17 Day Diet*
book to learn about all my strategies for overcoming barriers. Which
ones can you apply today?

_____

_____

_____

_____

_____

_____

_____

DAY 13—MY DAILY FOOD CHART   DATE

Dr. Mike's Food Tip of the Day

More and more restaurants are providing calorie and nutrition information about items on their menus—even the major fast-food chains.
Some have special sections of the menu devoted to low-fat, reduced-
calorie healthy choices for their dieting diners. Seek them out so you
can eat out without guilt!

WEIGHT

WATER INTAKE

number of 8-ounce glasses

☐ ☐ ☐ ☐
☐ ☐ ☐ ☐

FOOD INTAKE

number of servings

☐ Lean Proteins

☐ Cleansing
    Vegetables

☐ Natural Starch/
    High-Fiber
    Cereal/or Pasta
    (2 servings)

☐ Fruit
    (2 servings)

☐ Probiotic Foods/
    Dairy/Dairy Subs
    (1–2 servings)

☐ Friendly Fats
    (1–2 tablespoons)

☐ Optional Snack

Breakfast

Lunch

Dinner

Snacks

Dr. Mike's Workout Tip of the Day

A family member is hospitalized. There is a death in the family. You've had surgery or sustained a serious injury. There are going to be situations in life that may prevent you from exercising for sustained periods of time. When the crisis has passed, start slowly. Try to get in 17 minutes of gentle exercise, just as you did when you began the 17 Day Diet.

Cardio

DATE	ACTIVITY DESCRIPTION	DURATION	CALORIES BURNED	DISTANCE	STEPS

Toning Exercises

EXERCISES	SETS	REPS	WEIGHT	TIME	CALORIES BURNED

DAY 13—MY DAILY JOURNAL

What worked well?

_____

_____

_____

What didn't work well?

_____

_____

_____

I experienced the following challenges:

_____

_____

_____

Ways to overcome these challenges
(brainstorm as many problem-solvers as you can):

_____

_____

_____

From your list, choose the best solutions and develop
strategies for success.

_____

_____

_____

Reflections: Journal how you're feeling, your successes, anything that
comes to mind about your progress so far. Read through *The 17 Day Diet*
book to learn about all my strategies for overcoming barriers. Which
ones can you apply today?

_____

_____

_____

_____

_____

_____

DAY 14—MY DAILY FOOD CHART   DATE

Dr. Mike's Food Tip of the Day

Stop! If you step on the scale this weekend and see you have gained 3, 4, or 5 pounds (no more!), it's time to put on the brakes. To get back to your goal weight fastest, go back to the Accelerate Cycle. To maintain top-of-mind awareness about your weight, record it every week. You've worked too hard to let 5 pounds become 10, then 20!

WEIGHT

WATER INTAKE
number of 8-ounce glasses

☐ ☐ ☐ ☐
☐ ☐ ☐ ☐

FOOD INTAKE
number of servings

☐ Lean Proteins

☐ Cleansing
Vegetables

☐ Natural Starch/
High-Fiber
Cereal/or Pasta
(2 servings)

☐ Fruit
(2 servings)

☐ Probiotic Foods/
Dairy/Dairy Subs
(1–2 servings)

☐ Friendly Fats
(1–2 tablespoons)

☐ Optional Snack

Breakfast

Lunch

Dinner

Snacks

Dr. Mike's Workout Tip of the Day

Incorporating strength-training into your workout routine is equally important when it comes to staying healthy and keeping the muscles strong. Alternate the days on which you focus on strength-training and cardiovascular exercise. Working out with weights helps increase metabolism, burn calories, and tone and sculpt your muscles.

Cardio

DATE	ACTIVITY DESCRIPTION	DURATION	CALORIES BURNED	DISTANCE	STEPS

Toning Exercises

EXERCISES	SETS	REPS	WEIGHT	TIME	CALORIES BURNED

DAY 14—MY DAILY JOURNAL

What worked well?

_____

_____

_____

What didn't work well?

_____

_____

_____

I experienced the following challenges:

_____

_____

_____

Ways to overcome these challenges
(brainstorm as many problem-solvers as you can):

_____

_____

_____

From your list, choose the best solutions and develop
strategies for success.

_____

_____

_____

Reflections: Journal how you're feeling, your successes, anything that comes to mind about your progress so far. Read through *The 17 Day Diet* book to learn about all my strategies for overcoming barriers. Which ones can you apply today?

_____

_____

_____

_____

_____

_____

DAY 15—MY DAILY FOOD CHART   DATE

Dr. Mike's Food Tip of the Day

Restaurant go-to meals: Menus can be overwhelming unless you mentally prepare yourself for what you will and won't order when dining out. Look for grilled or baked chicken dishes (without cream sauces); grilled, baked, or blackened fish; steamed veggies; rice; baked white or sweet potato; salad with light dressing on the side; and broth-based soups.

WEIGHT

WATER INTAKE

number of 8-ounce glasses

☐ ☐ ☐ ☐
☐ ☐ ☐ ☐

FOOD INTAKE

number of servings

☐ Lean Proteins

☐ Cleansing
    Vegetables

☐ Natural Starch/
    High-Fiber
    Cereal/or Pasta
    (2 servings)

☐ Fruit
    (2 servings)

☐ Probiotic Foods/
    Dairy/Dairy Subs
    (1–2 servings)

☐ Friendly Fats
    (1–2 tablespoons)

☐ Optional Snack

Breakfast

_____
_____
_____
_____
_____

Lunch

_____
_____
_____
_____

Dinner

_____
_____
_____
_____

Snacks

_____
_____

Dr. Mike's Workout Tip of the Day

Be a kid again! Playing with your kids . . . or playing *like* a kid is one way to keep moving in a different way. Have a Hula-Hoop contest with them to see who can keep theirs going the longest. Skip down the sidewalk with your child. Climb the jungle gym with him or her at the playground, then try out the suspended rings. Climb a tree. You get the idea . . . It can be recess anytime you want it to be!

Cardio

DATE	ACTIVITY DESCRIPTION	DURATION	CALORIES BURNED	DISTANCE	STEPS

Toning Exercises

EXERCISES	SETS	REPS	WEIGHT	TIME	CALORIES BURNED

DAY 15—MY DAILY JOURNAL

What worked well?

_____
_____
_____

What didn't work well?

_____
_____
_____

I experienced the following challenges:

_____
_____
_____

Ways to overcome these challenges
(brainstorm as many problem-solvers as you can):

_____
_____
_____

From your list, choose the best solutions and develop
strategies for success.

_____
_____
_____

Reflections: Journal how you're feeling, your successes, anything that
comes to mind about your progress so far. Read through *The 17 Day Diet*
book to learn about all my strategies for overcoming barriers. Which
ones can you apply today?

_____
_____
_____
_____
_____
_____

DAY 16—MY DAILY FOOD CHART   DATE

Dr. Mike's Food Tip of the Day

Low-fat and fat-free foods aren't always a healthy choice, since many of them are high in sugar and calories. Check the ingredients list, and be aware that ingredients are listed in the order they are present in the product. If sugar or high-fructose corn syrup is at the top of the ingredients list, that food is not a healthy choice!

WEIGHT

WATER INTAKE

number of 8-ounce glasses

☐ ☐ ☐ ☐
☐ ☐ ☐ ☐

FOOD INTAKE

number of servings

☐ Lean Proteins

☐ Cleansing Vegetables

☐ Natural Starch/ High-Fiber Cereal/or Pasta (2 servings)

☐ Fruit (2 servings)

☐ Probiotic Foods/ Dairy/Dairy Subs (1–2 servings)

☐ Friendly Fats (1–2 tablespoons)

☐ Optional Snack

Breakfast

_____

_____

_____

_____

_____

Lunch

_____

_____

_____

_____

_____

Dinner

_____

_____

_____

_____

Snacks

_____

_____

Dr. Mike's Workout Tip of the Day

Tai chi, a gentle, flowing martial arts form that originated in China, may be a nice adjunct to your current fitness program. While it won't increase your aerobic fitness, studies show it can help lower blood pressure, boost the immune system, relieve stress, and increase flexibility, strength, and balance. If tai chi classes aren't available in your area, look for a tai chi DVD to use at home.

Cardio

DATE	ACTIVITY DESCRIPTION	DURATION	CALORIES BURNED	DISTANCE	STEPS

Toning Exercises

EXERCISES	SETS	REPS	WEIGHT	TIME	CALORIES BURNED

DAY 16—MY DAILY JOURNAL

What worked well?

_____
_____
_____

What didn't work well?

_____
_____
_____

I experienced the following challenges:

_____
_____
_____

Ways to overcome these challenges
(brainstorm as many problem-solvers as you can):

_____
_____
_____

From your list, choose the best solutions and develop
strategies for success.

_____
_____
_____

Reflections: Journal how you're feeling, your successes, anything that
comes to mind about your progress so far. Read through *The 17 Day Diet*
book to learn about all my strategies for overcoming barriers. Which
ones can you apply today?

_____
_____
_____
_____
_____
_____
_____

DAY 17—MY DAILY FOOD CHART   DATE

Dr. Mike's Food Tip of the Day

Watching your weight and what you eat, day to day, gets easier as you settle into the foods you'll shop for each week, the meals you'll prepare, and the items you'll avoid or limit to the weekends. Breathe a sigh of relief. Your new lifestyle of healthy eating and physical activity becomes a life of ease. You have indeed arrived!

WEIGHT

WATER INTAKE

number of 8-ounce glasses

☐ ☐ ☐ ☐
☐ ☐ ☐ ☐

FOOD INTAKE

number of servings

☐ Lean Proteins

☐ Cleansing Vegetables

☐ Natural Starch/ High-Fiber Cereal/or Pasta (2 servings)

☐ Fruit (2 servings)

☐ Probiotic Foods/ Dairy/Dairy Subs (1–2 servings)

☐ Friendly Fats (1–2 tablespoons)

☐ Optional Snack

Breakfast

_____
_____
_____
_____
_____

Lunch

_____
_____
_____
_____

Dinner

_____
_____
_____
_____

Snacks

_____
_____

Dr. Mike's Workout Tip of the Day

For many of you, *exercise* used to be a dirty word that you rarely used. You deceived yourself into thinking you enjoyed your couch-potato kind of life. Now look at yourself in the mirror and smile. The race isn't fully run, and there will be stumbles and even some falls, but I encourage you to persevere. Walk on! Run on! Your body is thanking you . . .

Cardio

DATE	ACTIVITY DESCRIPTION	DURATION	CALORIES BURNED	DISTANCE	STEPS

Toning Exercises

EXERCISES	SETS	REPS	WEIGHT	TIME	CALORIES BURNED

DAY 17—MY DAILY JOURNAL

What worked well?

_____

_____

_____

What didn't work well?

_____

_____

_____

I experienced the following challenges:

_____

_____

_____

Ways to overcome these challenges
(brainstorm as many problem-solvers as you can):

_____

_____

_____

From your list, choose the best solutions and develop
strategies for success.

_____

_____

_____

Reflections: Journal how you're feeling, your successes, anything that
comes to mind about your progress so far. Read through *The 17 Day Diet*
book to learn about all my strategies for overcoming barriers. Which
ones can you apply today?

_____

_____

_____

_____

_____

_____

_____

Review: Weight-Loss Checklist—Cycle 4

Can you relate to any of these?

1. Am I struggling with maintaining portion control?

    ☐ Always   ☐ Sometimes   ☐ Rarely or Never

2. Do I find myself binging on my trouble foods?

    ☐ Always   ☐ Sometimes   ☐ Rarely or Never

3. Do I feel myself losing motivation to keep off the weight I've lost?

    ☐ Always   ☐ Sometimes   ☐ Rarely or Never

4. Am I fully committed to incorporating physical exercise into my daily life . . . for the rest of my life?

    ☐ Always   ☐ Sometimes   ☐ Rarely or Never

5. Are there other obstacles I am struggling with to maintain my weight loss?

    ☐ Always   ☐ Sometimes   ☐ Rarely or Never

If so, list:

_____

_____

_____

_____

So far, I have lost _____ pounds.

The 17 Day Diet Maintenance Journal

....

Now that you have successfully reached your goal, it's time to look ahead to the rest of your life! Staying healthy, fit, and within 3 to 5 pounds of your goal weight is now your daily challenge. Take time to journal (at least) weekly about how you are maintaining your weight, any changes in weight you are experiencing, good and bad habits, etc.

Identify and evaluate weight changes

Are you weighing yourself at least weekly? ☐ Yes ☐ No

If there has been a weight gain, has it been recent or crept up gradually?

_____

_____

_____

_____

If your weight gain is more than 3 to 5 pounds above goal weight, ask yourself:

Have I changed my eating patterns? ☐ Yes ☐ No

Have I changed my activity level? ☐ Yes ☐ No

If you answered yes, can you identify bad habits that have contributed to these changes? If so, explain:

_____

_____

_____

_____

Are there other contributing factors (e.g., illness, medication changes, pregnancy)? If so, explain:

_____

_____

_____

_____

Action plan *(Check the actions you'll commit to, in order to get back on track.)*

☐ I will go back to Cycle 1 (Accelerate) or Cycle 2 (Activate) of the 17 Day Diet.

☐ I will begin recording my food intake.

☐ I will begin carefully policing my portions.

☐ I will restart or step up my physical activity.

Write in your own action:

_____

_____

_____

_____

Carefully think about answers to the following and record them under the headings below.

I do not want to regain the weight I have lost because:

1. _____

2. _____

3. _____

4. _____

I will strive daily to keep up the following healthy eating habits:

1. _____

2. _____

3. _____

4. _____

I will strive daily to keep up the following good exercise habits:

1. _____

2. _____

3. _____

4. _____

I must become more aware of the following areas of danger and self-sabotage:

1. _____

2. _____

3. _____

4. _____

The 17 Day Diet Shopping List

The eyes are the window to the soul, but the pantry and fridge? The gateway to a big gut—unless you stock them with care. When you're dieting, it's especially important to stock up on nutritious foods and not waste calories on high-fat "extras." It all starts in the supermarket, so to make shopping a real breeze, I've included a grocery list for the 17 Day Diet. It lists all of the important, high-nutrient foods you need for success. Grab a cart and let's go!

The Perimeter

The outside aisles of the supermarket, known as the perimeter, are where you will find the majority of foods you'll be enjoying on the 17 Day Diet. This is where the cleansing vegetables, fruits, lean proteins (meat, poultry, fish), and dairy are usually located.

The Produce Aisle

Vegetables

Dark, Leafy Greens

Alfalfa *(Cycles 3–4)*

Beet greens *(Cycles 1–4)*

Bok choy *(Cycles 3–4)*

Collard greens *(Cycles 1–4)*

Dandelion greens *(Cycles 3–4)*

Kale *(Cycles 1–4)*

Mustard greens *(Cycles 3–4)*

Spinach *(Cycles 1–4)*

Swiss chard *(Cycles 3–4)*

Turnip greens *(Cycles 1–4)*

Cruciferous Vegetables

Broccoli *(Cycles 1–4)*

Brussels sprouts *(Cycles 1–4)*

Cabbage *(Cycles 1–4)*

Cauliflower *(Cycles 1–4)*

Kohlrabi *(Cycles 3–4)*

Radishes *(Cycles 3–4)*

Sauerkraut *(Cycles 1–4) (Note: Sold in bags in the produce section. Also sold in cans and jars in interior aisles.)*

Roots and Tubers

Beets *(Cycles 3–4)*

Breadfruit *(Cycles 2–4)*

Carrots *(Cycles 1–4)*

Jerusalem artichoke *(Cycles 3–4)*

Jicama *(Cycles 3–4)*

Parsnips *(Cycles 3–4)*

Potatoes *(Cycles 2–4)*

Rutabaga *(Cycles 3–4)*

Sweet potatoes *(Cycles 2–4)*

Taro *(Cycles 2–4)*

Turnips *(Cycles 3–4)*

Yams *(Cycles 2–4)*

Salad Greens

Arugula *(Cycles 1–4)*

Cilantro *(Cycles 3–4)*

Endive *(Cycles 1–4)*

Escarole *(Cycles 1–4)*

Lettuce *(Cycles 1–4)*
- Boston/Bibb
- Iceberg
- Loose-leaf
- Romaine

Parsley *(Cycles 1–4)*

Radicchio *(Cycles 1–4)*

Watercress *(Cycles 1–4)*

Legumes

Beans, snap *(green)* *(Cycles 1–4)*

Beans, snap *(yellow wax)* *(Cycles 3–4)*

Fava beans *(Cycles 2–4)*

Peapods *(Cycles 3–4)*

Peas, shelled *(Cycles 2–4)*

Soybeans, fresh *(edamame)* *(Cycles 2–4)*

Mushrooms

Mushrooms *(Cycles 1–4)*
- Button
- Cremini
- Portobello
- Shiitake

Summer Squash

Chayote *(Cycles 3–4)*

Pattypan *(Cycles 3–4)*

Yellow squash *(Cycles 3–4)*

Zucchini *(Cycles 3–4)*

Winter Squash

Acorn squash *(Cycles 2–4)*

Butternut squash *(Cycles 2–4)*

Hubbard squash *(Cycles 2–4)*

Pumpkin squash *(Cycles 2–4)*

Spaghetti squash *(Cycles 2–4)*

Other Vegetables

Artichoke *(Cycles 1–4)*
Artichoke hearts *(Cycles 1–4)*
Asparagus *(Cycles 1–4)*
Bamboo shoots *(Cycles 3–4)*
Celery *(Cycles 1–4)*
Corn *(Cycles 2–4)*
Cucumbers *(Cycles 1–4)*
Eggplant *(Cycles 1–4)*
Fennel *(Cycles 3–4)*
Grape leaves *(Cycles 3–4)*
Kelp *(and other edible seaweeds)* *(Cycles 3–4)*
Okra *(Cycles 1–4)*
Peppers, chili *(Cycles 3–4)*

- Ancho
- Jalapeño
- Pasilla
- Serrano

Peppers, sweet *(Cycles 1–4)*

- Green bell
- Red bell
- Yellow bell

Tomatillos *(Cycles 1–4)*
Tomatoes *(Cycles 1–4)*

- Cherry
- Plum
- Red

Alliums

Garlic *(Cycles 1–4)*
Leeks *(Cycles 1–4)*
Onions *(Cycles 1–4)*
Scallions *(Cycles 1–4)*
Shallots *(Cycles 1–4)*

Soy-Based and Asian Foods

Tofu

(If you are a vegetarian, tofu can be one of your proteins on the 17 Day Diet.)
    Tempeh *(Cycles 1–4)*
    Tofu, firm *(Cycles 1–4)*
    Tofu hot dogs, bacon, and sausage links *(Cycles 1–4)*
    • Tofu bacon
    • Tofu bulk sausage
    • Tofu Canadian bacon
    • Tofu hot dogs
    • Tofu link sausage
    Tofu, soft *(Cycles 1–4)*
    Veggie burgers, crumbles, and meatballs *(Cycles 1–4)*
    • Burgers
    • Crumbles
    • Meatballs

Fruits

Berries

    Blackberries *(Cycles 1–4)*
    Blueberries *(Cycles 1–4)*
    Cranberries *(Cycles 1–4)*
    Currants *(Cycles 3–4)*
    Gooseberries *(Cycles 1–4)*
    Loganberries *(Cycles 1–4)*
    Raspberries *(Cycles 1–4)*
    Strawberries *(Cycles 1–4)*

Citrus Fruits

    Grapefruit *(Cycles 1–4)*
    Kumquats *(Cycles 3–4)*
    Lemons *(Cycles 3–4)*
    Limes *(Cycles 3–4)*
    Oranges *(Cycles 1–4)*

Tangelo *(Cycles 3–4)*

Tangerines *(Cycles 3–4)*

Melons

Cantaloupe *(Cycles 3–4)*

Honeydew melon *(Cycles 3–4)*

Watermelon *(Cycles 3–4)*

Tropical Fruits

Avocados, Hass *(Cycles 3–4)*

Bananas *(Cycles 3–4)*

Guava *(Cycles 3–4)*

Kiwi *(Cycles 3–4)*

Mango *(Cycles 3–4)*

Papaya *(Cycles 3–4)*

Pineapple *(Cycles 3–4)*

Plantains *(Cycles 3–4)*

Fruits with Pits

Apricots *(Cycles 3–4)*

Cherries *(Cycles 3–4)*

Nectarines *(Cycles 1–4)*

Peaches *(Cycles 1–4)*

Plums *(Cycles 1–4)*

Dried Fruits

Prunes *(Cycles 1–4)*

Grapes

Grapes
- Green *(Cycles 3–4)*
- Red *(Cycles 1–4)*

Other Fruits

Apples *(Cycles 1–4)*
Figs *(Cycles 3–4)*
Nopales *(prickly pear cactus) (Cycles 3–4)*
Pears *(Cycles 1–4)*
Pomegranates *(Cycles 3–4)*
Rhubarb *(Cycles 3–4)*

The Deli Counter

Only reduced-fat versions of cold cuts and deli meats are on the 17 Day Diet plan.

Cold Cuts/Deli Meats

Chicken breast, roasted *(Cycles 1–4)*
Turkey breast, roasted *(Cycles 1–4)*

The Fish Counter

Fresh Fish

Warm-Water Fish

Bass *(Cycles 1–4)*
Catfish *(Cycles 1–4)*
Cod *(Cycles 1–4)*
Flounder *(Cycles 1–4)*
Halibut *(Cycles 1–4)*
Monkfish *(Cycles 1–4)*
Perch *(Cycles 1–4)*
Pollock *(Cycles 1–4)*
Shad *(Cycles 1–4)*
Snapper *(Cycles 1–4)*
Tilapia *(Cycles 1–4)*

Cold-Water Fish

Bluefish *(Cycles 1–4)**

Haddock *(Cycles 1–4)*

Herring *(Cycles 1–4)*

Mackerel *(Cycles 1–4)*†

Mahimahi *(dolphin fish) (Cycles 1–4)*

Salmon *(Cycles 1–4)*

Sardines *(Cycles 1–4)*

Shark *(Cycles 1–4)*†

Sole *(Cycles 1–4)*

Swordfish *(Cycles 1–4)*†

Trout *(Cycles 1–4)*

Tuna *(bigeye, ahi) (Cycles 1–4)*†

Tuna *(canned albacore and yellowfin) (Cycles 1–4)**

Fresh Shellfish

Clams, cooked *(Cycles 2–4)*

Crabmeat, cooked *(Cycles 2–4)*

Lobster, steamed *(Cycles 2–4)*

Mussels, steamed *(Cycles 2–4)*

Oysters, raw *(Cycles 2–4)*

Scallops, raw *(Cycles 2–4)*

Shrimp, cooked *(Cycles 2–4)*

Squid, raw *(Cycles 2–4)*

Prepared Fish and Shellfish

Lox/Smoked Salmon *(Cycles 1–4)*

(For other fish you can eat on the 17 Day Diet, see the Food Guide on pages 301–314.)

---

*Fish with high levels of mercury (from 0.3 to 0.49 parts per million)
†Fish with highest levels of mercury (more than 0.5 parts per million) Sources: Food and Drug Administration; Environmental Protection Agency

The Meat Department

Beef

Flank steaks *(Cycles 2–4)*
Ground, lean *(Cycles 2–4)*
Round cuts *(Cycles 2–4)*
Sirloin cuts *(Cycles 2–4)*

Pork

Loin cuts *(Cycles 2–4)*
Sirloin cuts *(Cycles 2–4)*

Lamb

Loin *(Cycles 2–4)*
Shanks *(Cycles 2–4)*

Veal

Cutlets *(Cycles 2–4)*

Game

Beefalo *(Cycles 2–4)*
Buffalo *(Cycles 2–4)*
Venison *(Cycles 2–4)*

The Poultry Section

Chicken

Breast *(Cycles 1–4)*
Cornish hens *(Cycles 3–4)*

Turkey

Breast *(Cycles 1–4)*
Ground, lean *(Cycles 1–4)*

Game Birds

Ostrich *(Cycles 3–4)*
Pheasant *(Cycles 3–4)*
Quail *(Cycles 3–4)*

Sausage, Lunch Meats, and Cured Poultry (Reduced Fat Only)

Canadian bacon *(Cycles 3–4)*
Turkey bacon *(Cycles 3–4)*
Turkey ham *(Cycles 3–4)*
Turkey Italian sausage *(Cycles 3–4)*

The Dairy Case

Fresh Cheese

Breakstone's LivActive cottage cheese *(Cycles 1–4)*
Cottage cheese, low fat *(Cycles 3–4)*
Mozzarella, part skim *(Cycles 3–4)*
Ricotta, part skim *(Cycles 3–4)*

Soft and Semisoft Cheese (Low Fat Only)

Babybel low-fat cheese *(Cycles 3–4)*
Brie *(Cycles 3–4)*
Camembert *(Cycles 3–4)*
Edam *(Cycles 3–4)*
Feta *(Cycles 3–4)*
Goat *(Cycles 3–4)*
Limburger *(Cycles 3–4)*
String cheese *(Cycles 3–4)*

Hard and Semihard Cheese (Low Fat Only)

Cheddar *(Cycles 3–4)*

Fontina *(Cycles 3–4)*

Parmigiano-reggiano *(Cycles 3–4)*

Dips and Salsa

Salsa *(Cycles 1–4)*

Butter, Margarine, and Spreads

Cholesterol-lowering margarines *(Cycles 1–4)*

Milk

Lactaid, skim *(Cycles 3–4)*

Low-fat acidophilus milk *(Cycles 1–4)*

Low-fat buttermilk (1%) *(Cycles 3–4)*

Nonfat, skim *(Cycles 3–4)*

Reduced fat (2%) *(Cycles 3–4)*

Cream

Sour cream, fat-free *(Cycles 1–4)*

Soy Milk and Other Dairy Substitutes

Moo (Not!), low carb *(Cycles 3–4)*

Silk Soymilk, organic unsweetened *(Cycles 3–4)*

Sugar-free almond milk *(Cycles 3–4)*

Sugar-free rice milk *(Cycles 3–4)*

Sugar-free soy milk *(Cycles 3–4)*

Unsweetened soy milk, most brands *(Cycles 3–4)*

Soy Products

Miso, reduced salt *(Cycles 1–4)*

Tempeh *(Cycles 1–4)*

Yogurt and Other Cultured Foods

Greek yogurt *(0–2%) (Cycles 1–4)*

Kefir *(Cycles 1–4)*

Plain, low-fat, most brands *(Cycles 1–4)*

Plain, whole milk, most brands *(Cycles 1–4)*

Yakult (probiotic beverage) *(Cycles 1–4)*

Eggs

Egg substitutes *(Cycles 1–4)*

Egg whites *(Cycles 1–4)*

Eggs *(Cycles 1–4)*

THE INTERIOR

The interior aisles of the supermarket contain foods that do not require refrigeration. These include prepared, canned, and boxed foods, ranging from canned vegetables, fruits, and soups to boxed and/or packaged cereals, grains, and rice.

The Breakfast Foods Aisle

Cereal

Cold Cereal

All-Bran *(Cycles 3–4)*

All-Bran Bran Buds *(Cycles 3–4)*

Fiber One *(Cycles 3–4)*

Gluten-free cold cereals *(Cycles 3–4)*

Low-sugar granola *(Cycles 3–4)*

Post 100% Bran *(Cycles 3–4)*

Hot Cereal

Farina *(Cycles 2–4)*

Cream of Wheat *(Cycles 2–4)*

Oat bran *(Cycles 2–4)*

Irish oat bran *(Cycles 2–4)*

Irish oatmeal, steel cut *(Cycles 2–4)*

Instant whole-grain oatmeal *(Cycles 2–4)*

Instant oatmeal *(Cycles 2–4)*

Old-fashioned Oats, Quick *(Cycles 2–4)*

Grits, Quick *(Cycles 2–4)*

Wheatena *(Cycles 2–4)*

The Bread Aisle

Bread Products

Cracked wheat bread *(Cycles 3–4)*

Ezekiel bread *(Cycles 3–4)*

Fiber-enriched bread *(Cycles 3–4)*

Gluten-free bread *(Cycles 3–4)*

Multigrain bread *(Cycles 3–4)*

Oat bran bread *(Cycles 3–4)*

Pumpernickel bread *(Cycles 3–4)*

Rye bread *(Cycles 3–4)*

Sprouted grain bread *(Cycles 3–4)*

Sugar-free bread *(Cycles 3–4)*

Whole-wheat bread *(Cycles 3–4)*

Whole-wheat pita bread *(Cycles 3–4)*

Whole-wheat tortilla *(Cycles 3–4)*

Whole-wheat wraps *(Cycles 3–4)*

The Baking Aisle

For Cooking

These ingredients are sometimes used in my recipes in small amounts for baking and flavoring.

Baking soda *(Cycles 1–4)*

Cocoa powder, unsweetened *(Cycles 1–4)*

Cornstarch *(Cycles 1–4)*

Knox Gelatine, unflavored *(Cycles 1–4)*

Sugar Substitute

Truvia *(Cycles 1–4)*

The Condiments Aisle

Salad Dressings

Fat-free dressings *(Cycles 1–4)*

Reduced-calorie dressings *(Cycles 3–4)*

Reduced-fat dressings *(Cycles 3–4)*

Light dressings *(Cycles 3–4)*

Salad dressings *(Cycles 3–4)*

Oils and Vinegars

Canola oil *(Cycles 3–4)*

Flaxseed oil *(Cycles 1–4)*

Olive oil *(Cycles 1–4)*

Walnut oil *(Cycles 3–4)*

Balsamic vinegar *(Cycles 1–4)*

Cider vinegar *(Cycles 1–4)*

Rice vinegar *(Cycles 1–4)*

Wine vinegar *(Cycles 1–4)*

Seasoned rice vinegar *(Cycles 1–4)*

Mayonnaise

Mayonnaise, fat-free *(Cycles 1–4)*

Mayonnaise, light *(Cycles 3–4)*

Mayonnaise *(Cycles 3–4)*

Tartar Sauce

Tartar sauce, low fat *(Cycles 3–4)*

Mexican Condiments and Sauces

Salsa *(Cycles 1–4)*
Enchilada sauce *(Cycles 1–4)*
Taco sauce *(Cycles 1–4)*

Asian Condiments and Sauces

Soy sauce, lite *(Cycles 1–4)*
Teriyaki sauce *(Cycles 1–4)*
Wasabi, most brands *(Cycles 1–4)*
Kimchi (Korean cabbage) *(Cycles 1–4)*

Other Condiments

Bacon bits *(Cycles 1–4)*
- Hormel real bacon bits

Barbecue sauce, Walden Farms carb-free *(Cycles 1–4)*
Cocktail sauce *(Cycles 1–4)*
Clam juice, most brands *(Cycles 1–4)*
Horseradish *(Cycles 1–4)*
Hot sauce *(Cycles 1–4)*
- Hot sauce, most brands
- Tabasco sauce

Jams, jellies, and preserves *(Cycles 1–4)*
- No added sugar

Ketchup *(Cycles 1–4)*
- Reduced sugar

Mustard *(Cycles 1–4)*
- Chinese style
- Dijon
- Yellow

Pancake and flavored syrups *(Cycles 1–4)*
- Sugar-free

Steak sauce *(Cycles 1–4)*
- A1, original
- Lawry's Carb Options Steak Sauce

Sweet relish, sugar-free *(Cycles 1–4)*

Worcestershire sauce *(Cycles 1–4)*

The Canned and Jarred Foods Aisle

Canned and Jarred Beans and Legumes

Adzuki beans, most brands *(Cycles 2–4)*

Black beans, most brands *(Cycles 2–4)*

Black soybeans, Eden Organic and most brands *(Cycles 2–4)*

Black-eyed peas, most brands *(Cycles 2–4)*

Butter beans, most brands *(Cycles 2–4)*

Cannellini, most brands *(Cycles 2–4)*

Garbanzo beans (chickpeas), most brands *(Cycles 2–4)*

Great northern beans, most brands *(Cycles 2–4)*

Green split peas, most brands *(Cycles 2–4)*

Kidney beans, most brands *(Cycles 2–4)*

Lentils, most brands *(Cycles 2–4)*

Lima beans, baby, most brands *(Cycles 2–4)*

Navy beans, most brands *(Cycles 2–4)*

Peas, most brands *(Cycles 2–4)*

Pinto beans, most brands *(Cycles 2–4)*

Red lentils, most brands *(Cycles 2–4)*

Soybeans, most brands *(Cycles 2–4)*

White beans, most brands *(Cycles 2–4)*

Canned and Jarred Soups and Broth

Beef broth *(Cycles 1–4)*
- Fat-free beef broth

Chicken broth *(Cycles 1–4)*
- Fat-free chicken broth

Vegetable broth *(Cycles 1–4)*
- Fat-free vegetable broth

Canned and Jarred Vegetables and Fruit

Beets *(Cycles 3–4)*

Cut green beans *(Cycles 1–4)*

Pineapple, canned in its own juice *(Cycles 3–4)*

Sauerkraut, canned or jarred *(Cycles 1–4)*

Canned Seafood

Baby clams *(Cycles 2–4)*

Clams, chopped or minced *(Cycles 2–4)*

Crabmeat, fancy white *(Cycles 2–4)*

Crabmeat, lump *(Cycles 2–4)*

Mackerel, most brands *(Cycles 2–4)*

Mussels, smoked *(Cycles 2–4)*

Oysters, smoked *(Cycles 2–4)*

Salmon, all varieties, most brands *(Cycles 1–4)*

Sardines, in tomato sauce *(Cycles 1–4)*

Sardines, in water *(Cycles 1–4)*

Shrimp, medium *(Cycles 2–4)*

Shrimp, tiny *(Cycles 2–4)*

Tuna, albacore (in water) *(Cycles 1–4)*

Tuna, chunk (in water) *(Cycles 1–4)*

Tuna, light (in water) *(Cycles 1–4)*

Canned and Jarred Tomatoes

Tomatoes, crushed, with Italian herbs *(Cycles 1–4)*

Tomatoes, diced *(Cycles 1–4)*

Tomatoes, pureed *(Cycles 1–4)*

Tomatoes, stewed *(Cycles 1–4)*

Tomatoes, stewed, Italian style *(Cycles 1–4)*

**Canned and Jarred Tomato and Pasta Sauces/
Tomato Paste**

Low-carb marinara sauce *(no sugar added) (Cycles 1–4)*
Marinara sauce, no sugar added *(Cycles 1–4)*
Tomato paste *(Cycles 1–4)*

The Pasta, Grains, Beans, and Legumes Aisle

Whole Grains

Amaranth *(Cycles 2–4)*
Barley, pearled *(Cycles 2–4)*
Buckwheat groats *(kasha) (Cycles 2–4)*
Bulgur *(Cycles 2–4)*
Couscous, whole wheat *(Cycles 2–4)*
Millet *(Cycles 2–4)*
Oats *(Cycles 2–4)*
Rice, brown *(Cycles 2–4)*
Rice, long grain *(basmati) (Cycles 2–4)*
Rice, wild *(Cycles 2–4)*

Dried Beans and Legumes

Adzuki *(Cycles 2–4)*
Black beans *(Cycles 2–4)*
Black-eyed peas *(Cycles 2–4)*
Cannellini *(white kidney beans) (Cycles 2–4)*
Chickpeas *(garbanzo beans) (Cycles 2–4)*
Cranberry beans *(Roman) (Cycles 2–4)*
Fava *(broad bean) (Cycles 2–4)*
Great northern beans *(Cycles 2–4)*
Lentils *(Cycles 2–4)*
Lima beans, baby *(Cycles 2–4)*
Lima beans, large *(Cycles 2–4)*

Navy beans *(Cycles 2–4)*

Pink beans *(Cycles 2–4)*

Pinto beans *(Cycles 2–4)*

Red kidney beans *(Cycles 2–4)*

Soybeans *(Cycles 2–4)*

Split peas *(Cycles 2–4)*

Pasta

Gluten-free pasta *(Cycles 3–4)*

High-fiber pasta *(Cycles 3–4)*

Shirataki pasta *(Cycles 3–4)*

Soba noodles *(Cycles 3–4)*

Vegetable-based pasta *(Cycles 3–4)*

Whole-wheat pasta *(Cycles 3–4)*
- Angel hair
- Bow tie
- Penne
- *Radiatori*
- Shells
- Spaghetti
- Spirals

Whole-wheat spinach egg noodles *(Cycles 3–4)*

Udon noodles *(Cycles 3–4)*

The Snacks Aisle

Gelatin Mixes

Jell-O, sugar-free, all flavors *(Cycles 1–4)*

Pudding Mixes

Jell-O pudding and pie filling
- Cook and serve, sugar-free, vanilla, chocolate *(Cycles 2–4)*

- Instant, sugar-free, fat-free, vanilla, chocolate *(Cycles 2–4)*
- Pudding cup, sugar-free *(Cycles 3–4)*

Savory Snacks

Popcorn, microwave, light *(Cycles 3–4)*

Nuts and Seeds

Almonds, roasted, salted *(Cycles 3–4)*
Brazil nuts *(Cycles 3–4)*
Cashews *(Cycles 3–4)*
Hazelnuts *(Cycles 3–4)*
Macadamia nuts, roasted, salted *(Cycles 3–4)*
Mixed nuts *(Cycles 3–4)*
Peanuts, cocktail *(Cycles 3–4)*
Peanuts, dry roasted *(Cycles 3–4)*
Pecans *(Cycles 3–4)*
Pine nuts *(Cycles 3–4)*
Pistachios, dry roasted, salted in shell *(Cycles 3–4)*
Pumpkin seeds *(Cycles 3–4)*
Soybean nuts *(Cycles 3–4)*
Sunflower seeds, roasted, salted *(Cycles 3–4)*
Walnuts *(Cycles 3–4)*

The Beverage Aisle

Hot Drinks

Decaf black tea *(Cycles 1–4)*
Decaf coffee *(Cycles 1–4)*
Green tea *(Cycles 1–4)*
Herbal tea *(Cycles 1–4)*

The Frozen Foods Aisle

. . . .

Vegetables

Artichoke hearts, most brands *(Cycles 1–4)*

Asparagus spears, most brands *(Cycles 1–4)*

Broccoli, most brands *(Cycles 1–4)*

Brussels sprouts, most brands *(Cycles 1–4)*

Butternut squash, most brands *(Cycles 2–4)*

Carrots, most brands *(Cycles 1–4)*

Cauliflower, most brands *(Cycles 1–4)*

Collard greens, most brands *(Cycles 1–4)*

Corn, most brands *(Cycles 3–4)*

Corn, white, most brands *(Cycles 3–4)*

Green beans, most brands *(Cycles 1–4)*

Kale, most brands *(Cycles 1–4)*

Lima beans, baby, most brands *(Cycles 3–4)*

Lima beans, Fordhook, most brands *(Cycles 3–4)*

Okra, most brands *(Cycles 1–4)*

Peas, green, most brands *(Cycles 2–4)*

Peas, petite, most brands *(Cycles 2–4)*

Rutabaga, most brands *(Cycles 3–4)*

Spinach, most brands *(Cycles 1–4)*

Succotash, most brands *(Cycles 3–4)*

Summer squash, most brands *(Cycles 3–4)*

Turnip greens, most brands *(Cycles 1–4)*

Winter squash, most brands *(Cycles 1–4)*

Fruits

Blackberries, most brands, unsweetened *(Cycles 1–4)*

Blueberries, most brands, unsweetened *(Cycles 1–4)*

Mixed berries, most brands, unsweetened *(Cycles 1–4)*

Mixed fruits, most brands, unsweetened *(Cycles 3–4)*

Papaya chunks, most brands, unsweetened *(Cycles 3–4)*

Peaches, most brands, unsweetened *(Cycles 1–4)*
Raspberries, most brands, unsweetened *(Cycles 1–4)*
Strawberries, sliced, most brands, unsweetened *(Cycles 1–4)*
Strawberries, whole, most brands, unsweetened *(Cycles 1–4)*

Ice Cream and Desserts

Breyers CarbSmart, vanilla, chocolate *(Cycles 3–4)*
Breyers Smooth & Dreamy No Sugar Added ice cream, vanilla
(Cycles 3–4)
Dole Fruit Bars, all flavors *(Cycles 3–4)*
Edy's No Sugar Added ice cream, most flavors *(Cycles 3–4)*

Ice Cream Novelties

Blue Bunny Sweet Freedom Novelties, Almond Bar *(Cycles 3–4)*
Blue Bunny Sweet Freedom Novelties, no sugar added Vanilla
Fudge, Fudge Lite bar *(Cycles 3–4)*
Fudgsicle, 100 calorie Bar *(Cycles 3–4)*
100 Calorie Klondike ice cream bar *(Cycles 3–4)*
100 Calorie Klondike ice cream fudge bar *(Cycles 3–4)*
Skinny Cow ice cream sandwich *(Cycles 3–4)*

17 Brand-New Recipes from Dr. Mike

Smoothies

Peachy Shake

> 1 cup almond milk
> ½ cup frozen peaches
> ¼ cup raw instant oatmeal

With the addition of oatmeal, this shake makes a delicious, complete meal. Place all ingredients in a blender and blend until smooth. Use on Cycles 3–4.

Yield: 1 serving

Piña Colada Shake

> ½ cup silken tofu
> 1 cup almond milk
> ½ cup crushed pineapple
> ½ frozen banana
> 2 packets Truvia
> ½ teaspoon coconut extract

Place all ingredients in a blender and blend until smooth. Use on Cycles 3–4.

Yield: 1 large serving

Snacks, Sides, and Salads

Yummus

    2 cups cooked peas, drained

    ¼ cup water

    1 teaspoon crushed garlic

    1 small onion, chopped coarsely

    1 tablespoon olive oil

    1 tablespoon lemon juice

    ½ cup grated parmigiano-reggiano cheese

    ½ teaspoon kosher salt

    ½ teaspoon black pepper

Place all ingredients in a blender. Pulse until mixture is smooth but not pureed. Add a little bit more water if needed. Transfer to a serving bowl. Serve with fresh diced veggies. Use on Cycles 2–4.

Yield: 4 servings

Yogurt Cheese

    32 ounces fat-free Greek yogurt

    Spices (kosher salt, garlic powder, oregano)

Line a strainer with a coffee filter or white paper towel. Place the strainer over a bowl to catch the liquid. Spoon in 32 ounces of fat-free Greek yogurt. Cover and refrigerate for eight hours or overnight. Makes about 16 ounces of yogurt cheese. Mix in your favorite spices for a tangy dip for vegetables or as a topping for baked potatoes. Use on Cycles 1–4.

Yield: 5 servings

Green Bean Casserole

1 can (10.75 ounces) low-fat condensed cream of
   mushroom soup
¼ cup low-fat milk
1 teaspoon soy sauce
¼ teaspoon fresh ground pepper
2 14.5-ounce cans of French-style green beans, drained
3 tablespoons bacon bits or chips
1 medium onion, chopped
1 tablespoon olive oil

In a 1½-quart casserole dish, combine soup, milk, soy sauce, and pepper. Mix well. Add beans. Sprinkle bacon bits over the casserole.

In a small saucepan, cook onion in olive oil on high heat, until onion is brown. Place browned onions over the top of the casserole.

Bake at 350 degrees for 25 minutes. Use on Cycles 1–4.

Yield: 4 servings

Leek and Tomato Soup

2 tablespoons olive oil
3 medium leeks, sliced up to the green parts
1 tablespoon minced garlic
½ teaspoon salt
14-ounce can diced tomatoes
3 cups vegetable juice (V8)
1 teaspoon dried marjoram
¼ teaspoon fresh ground pepper

Heat oil in a large soup pot. Sauté leeks, garlic, and salt until leeks are soft. Slowly stir in tomatoes, vegetable juice, marjoram, and pepper. Cover and cook on low heat for 20 minutes. Use on Cycles 1–4.

Yield: 4 servings

17 Day Slimming Soup

3 cups cabbage, chopped
2 yellow squashes, chopped
1 large onion, chopped
3 large celery stalks with leaves, chopped
2 15-ounce cans crushed tomatoes
3 14-ounce cans fat-free chicken broth
1 cup vegetable juice
3 teaspoons salt
¼ teaspoon pepper

Place all ingredients in a large pan and simmer for one hour, or until vegetables are soft. Use on Cycles 1–4.

Yield: 16 servings

Ambrosia

1 20-ounce can crushed pineapple in 100% pineapple juice
1 8.25-ounce can lite fruit cocktail in pear juice, drained
1 1-ounce package instant sugar-free, fat-free pistachio
    pudding mix
1 tablespoon lemon juice
1½ cup sugar-free or fat-free whipped topping

In a large bowl, pour pineapple with its juice. Stir in the drained fruit cocktail and mix well. Stir in the powdered pudding mix and blend well. Fold in the lemon juice and whipped topping and blend well. Refrigerate for at least four hours prior to serving. Use on Cycles 3–4.

Yield: 8 servings

Main Meals
· · · · · · · · · · · · · · · · ·

Oven-Fried Cajun Tilapia

1 pound fresh tilapia—4 fillets
2 cups whole-wheat panko bread crumbs
1 teaspoon Cajun seasoning
½ teaspoon kosher salt
1½ cups low-fat buttermilk
Vegetable cooking spray

Spread bread crumbs out on a large platter. Sprinkle with Cajun seasoning and salt. Distribute spices evenly among bread crumbs. Fill a shallow bowl with the buttermilk. Dip each fillet in the buttermilk, then coat the fillet with bread crumbs. Place coated fillets on a baking pan or cookie sheet that has been coated with vegetable cooking spray. Then spray each fillet with the vegetable cooking spray. Bake fish in a 400-degree oven for 10–12 minutes or until fish flakes easily with a fork. Do not overcook. Use on Cycles 3–4.

Yield: 4 servings

Meat and Rice Loaf

1 cup cooked brown and wild rice
1 pound extra-lean ground beef
1 egg, beaten
1 medium onion, chopped
1 teaspoon salt
¼ teaspoon garlic powder
½ teaspoon dry mustard
½ teaspoon ground sage
1 tablespoon Worcestershire sauce

Mix all ingredients together and form into a loaf. Bake at 350 degrees for an hour and a half. Use on Cycles 2–4.

Yield: 4 servings

BBQ Chicken

4 chicken breasts
1 cup fat-free Catalina salad dressing
2 tablespoons teriyaki sauce
2 tablespoons lite soy sauce
1 tablespoon carb-free barbecue sauce (Walden Farms)

To make the marinade, combine salad dressing, teriyaki sauce, lite soy sauce, and barbecue sauce. Pour over chicken breasts and let marinade for at least three hours in the refrigerator. Grill or bake chicken breasts to desired doneness, basting occasionally with marinade. Use on Cycles 1–4.

Yield: 4 servings

Herbed Pork Chops

4 lean pork chops (about 4 to 5 ounces each), all visible fat
trimmed
2 sprigs fresh rosemary (chopped leaves)
1 tablespoon minced garlic
2 tablespoons olive oil

Using medium-low heat, sauté rosemary and garlic in olive oil until spices are soft. Add the pork chops. Cook well on both sides. Salt lightly before serving. Use on Cycles 1–4.

Yield: 4 servings

Scallops Kebab

1 pound scallops, raw
1 medium red bell pepper
1 medium green bell pepper
1 medium yellow bell pepper
8 white pearl onions
½ cup fat-free Italian salad dressing

Cut peppers into large chunks. Arrange scallops, pepper chunks, and onions on kebab skewers. Baste with vinaigrette and grill over a medium flame for about 20 minutes, brushing with remaining dressing. (Reduced-fat dressing may be used in place of vinaigrette.) Use on Cycles 1–4.

Yield: 4 servings

Super Stuffed Red Peppers

4 large red bell peppers

1 pound ground turkey

1 medium onion, chopped

2 medium tomatoes, chopped

½ cup chopped pecans

1 cup shiitake mushrooms, chopped

1 cup cooked bulgur wheat

1 tablespoon fresh basil

1 teaspoon red pepper

1 teaspoon kosher salt

¼ teaspoon black pepper

Cut out tops of red peppers and remove seed cores. Boil peppers in a large saucepan of water until just tender. Drain on a paper towel.

Brown turkey; drain any fat. Add onion, tomatoes, pecans, mushrooms, wheat, and spices. Sauté until all vegetables are soft. Stuff peppers with mixture and bake at 350 degrees for 30 minutes. Use on Cycles 3–4.

Yield: 4 servings

Mexican Bean Stew

2 tablespoons olive oil

1 tablespoon chopped garlic

1 medium onion, chopped

1 green bell pepper, chopped

2 15-ounce cans kidney beans, drained

1 15-ounce can of corn, drained

1 4-ounce can green chiles
2 28-ounce cans crushed tomatoes
1 packet taco seasoning mix

In a large saucepan, sauté garlic, onion, and green pepper in the olive oil until tender. Add the rest of the ingredients and bring to a simmer. With the lid on, simmer for 20 minutes. Use on Cycles 3–4.

Yield: 4 servings

Frozen Treats

Super-Strawberry Frozen Yogurt

2 6-ounce cartons of light fat-free strawberry yogurt
2 tablespoons Smuckers sugar-free strawberry jam

Mix together yogurt and jam. Blend well. Refrigerate for a few hours until mixture is very cold. I use a Hamilton Beach Ice Cream Maker, which makes 12 ounces of frozen yogurt at a time. Pour the mixture into the freezer bowl. Turn the motor on, and your dessert should be ready within 10 minutes.

Yield: 2 servings

Chocolaty Frozen Yogurt

12-ounces 2% Greek yogurt
1 tablespoon low-fat buttermilk
1 tablespoon agave nectar
2 teaspoons unsweetened baking cocoa
¼ cup Nestlé Quik sugar-free hot cocoa mix
½ teaspoon instant espresso powder
½ teaspoon vanilla extract

Combine the above ingredients. Mix well using a whisk. Refrigerate for a few hours until mixture is very cold. Pour the mixture into the freezer bowl. Turn the motor on, and your dessert should be ready within 15 to 20 minutes.

Yield: 2 servings

Exercise, Sports, and Everyday Activities Chart

● ●

You're burning calories reading this, even if you're not huffing through a treadmill workout at the same time. Stand up and read, and you'll fry even more calories. The point is, there's a lot of calorie-burning activity in any kind of motion, even sex. And the more calories you burn during the day, the more fat you lose. To give you a comprehensive look at which activities will torch the most calories, the chart below is adapted from the American College of Sports Medicine's *ACSM's Resource Manual for Guidelines for Exercise Testing and Prescription.*

To ratchet up your calorie-burning, look for ways to increase movement in your daily routine. This chart can help you. Also, use it to log your calorie-burning in this journal.

Calories burned per hour (for people of varying body weights)

EXERCISE	130 lb	155 lb	180 lb	205 lb
Aerobics, low impact	295	352	409	465
Aerobics, high impact	413	493	572	651
Aerobics, step	502	598	695	791
Aerobics, general	384	457	531	605
Aerobics class, instructing	354	422	490	558
Ballet, jazz, tap	266	317	368	419
Ballroom dancing, slow	177	211	245	279
Ballroom dancing, fast	325	387	449	512
Calisthenics, vigorous, push-ups, sit-ups	472	563	654	745
Calisthenics, light	207	246	286	326
Circuit training, minimal rest	472	563	654	745
Cycling, mountain bike, BMX	502	598	695	791
Cycling, <10 mph, leisure bicycling	236	281	327	372
Cycling, >20 mph, racing	944	1126	1308	1489
Cycling, 10–11.9 mph, light	354	422	490	558
Cycling, 12–13.9 mph, moderate	472	563	654	745
Cycling, 14–15.9 mph, vigorous	590	704	817	931
Jazzercise	354	422	490	558
Jumping rope, fast	708	844	981	1117
Jumping rope, moderate	590	704	817	931
Jumping rope, slow	472	563	654	745
Martial arts, judo, karate, jujitsu	590	704	817	931
Martial arts, kickboxing	590	704	817	931
Martial arts, tae kwon do	590	704	817	931
Rowing machine, light	207	246	286	326
Rowing machine, moderate	413	493	572	651
Rowing machine, vigorous	502	598	695	791
Running, 5 mph (12-minute mile)	472	563	654	745
Running, 5.2 mph (11.5-minute mile)	531	633	735	838
Running, 6 mph (10-minute mile)	590	704	817	931
Running, 6.7 mph (9-minute mile)	649	774	899	1024
Running, general	472	563	654	745
Ski machine	413	493	572	651
Stair machine	531	633	735	838
Stationary cycling, very light	177	211	245	279
Stationary cycling, light	325	387	449	512
Stationary cycling, moderate	413	493	572	651
Stationary cycling, vigorous	620	739	858	977
Swimming laps, freestyle, fast	590	704	817	931

EXERCISE (cont.)	130 lb	155 lb	180 lb	205 lb
Swimming laps, freestyle, slow	413	493	572	651
Swimming backstroke	413	493	572	651
Swimming breaststroke	590	704	817	931
Swimming butterfly	649	774	899	1024
Swimming leisurely, not laps	354	422	490	558
Swimming sidestroke	472	563	654	745
Walking, under 2.0 mph, very slow	118	141	163	186
Walking, 2.0 mph, slow	148	176	204	233
Walking, 2.5 mph	177	211	245	279
Walking, 3.0 mph, moderate	195	232	270	307
Walking, 3.5 mph, brisk pace	224	267	311	354
Walking, 3.5 mph, uphill	354	422	490	558
Water aerobics	236	281	327	372
Water jogging	472	563	654	745
Weight lifting, body building, vigorous	354	422	490	558
Weight lifting, light workout	177	211	245	279
Yoga	236	281	327	372
SPORTS	130 lb	155 lb	180 lb	205 lb
Archery	207	246	286	326
Backpacking, hiking with pack	413	493	572	651
Badminton	266	317	368	419
Basketball game, competitive	472	563	654	745
Basketball, noncompetitive	354	422	490	558
Billiards	148	176	204	233
Bowling	177	211	245	279
Boxing, punching bag	354	422	490	558
Boxing, sparring	531	633	735	838
Canoeing, camping trip	236	281	327	372
Canoeing, rowing, light	177	211	245	279
Canoeing, rowing, moderate	413	493	572	651
Canoeing, rowing, vigorous	708	844	981	1117
Croquet	148	176	204	233
Cross-country skiing, slow	413	493	572	651
Cross-country skiing, moderate	472	563	654	745
Cross-country skiing, vigorous	531	633	735	838
Darts (wall or lawn)	148	176	204	233
Downhill skiing, light	295	352	409	465
Downhill skiing, moderate	354	422	490	558
Downhill skiing, racing	472	563	654	745
Fencing	354	422	490	558

SPORTS (cont.)	130 lb	155 lb	180 lb	205 lb
Football, touch, flag, general	472	563	654	745
Frisbee playing, general	177	211	245	279
Golf, general	266	317	368	419
Golf, walking and carrying clubs	266	317	368	419
Golf, driving range	177	211	245	279
Golf, miniature golf	177	211	245	279
Golf, walking and pulling clubs	254	303	351	400
Golf, using power cart	207	246	286	326
Hacky sack	236	281	327	372
Handball	708	844	981	1117
Hiking, cross-country	354	422	490	558
Ice skating, average speed	413	493	572	651
Kayaking	295	352	409	465
Orienteering	531	633	735	838
Racquetball	413	493	572	651
Race walking	384	457	531	605
Riding a horse, general	236	281	327	372
Rock climbing, mountain climbing	472	563	654	745
Roller-skating	413	493	572	651
Rollerblading, in-line skating	708	844	981	1117
Sailing, yachting, ocean sailing	177	211	245	279
Shuffleboard, lawn bowling	177	211	245	279
Skateboarding	295	352	409	465
Skiing, water-skiing	354	422	490	558
Skimobiling	413	493	572	651
Skin diving, scuba diving	413	493	572	651
Sledding, tobogganing, luge	413	493	572	651
Snorkeling	295	352	409	465
Snowmobiling	207	246	286	326
Snowshoeing	472	563	654	745
Surfing, bodysurfing, or board surfing	177	211	245	279
Softball or baseball	295	352	409	465
Squash	708	844	981	1117
Table tennis, Ping-Pong	236	281	327	372
Tai chi	236	281	327	372
Tennis, doubles	354	422	490	558
Tennis, singles	472	563	654	745
Track and field (hurdles)	590	704	817	931
Trampoline	207	246	286	326
Volleyball, regular	177	211	245	279

SPORTS (cont.)	130 lb	155 lb	180 lb	205 lb
Volleyball, beach	472	563	654	745
Windsurfing, sailing	177	211	245	279
White-water rafting, kayaking, canoeing	295	352	409	465
EVERYDAY ACTIVITIES	130 lb	155 lb	180 lb	205 lb
Bird-watching	148	176	204	233
General housework	207	246	286	326
Cleaning gutters	295	352	409	465
Painting	266	317	368	419
Mowing lawn, walk, power mower	325	387	449	512
Mowing lawn, riding mower	148	176	204	233
Snowblower, walking	207	246	286	326
Snowblower, riding	177	211	245	279
Sex, foreplay	86	102	119	135
Sex, intercourse	250	298	346	394
Shoveling snow by hand	354	422	490	558
Raking lawn	254	303	351	400
Gardening, general	236	281	327	372
Standing, playing with children, light	165	197	229	261
Walking the dog	177	211	245	279
Walk/run, playing with children, moderate	236	281	327	372
Walk/run, playing with children, vigorous	295	352	409	465

The 17 Day Diet Food Guide

· ·

My Food Guide lists foods in alphabetical order so you'll have no trouble finding whatever you want to look up. Let's say, for example, you're looking for carrots. Go down to the C foods, and you'll find carrots listed there.

Each food entry lists the following information in this order: food item, serving size, calories. It then lists the amount of each of the following in grams: total fat, protein, carbohydrates, and fiber. The last column designates the cycle on which you can eat the particular food.

This guide, derived from the USDA National Nutrient Database, provides you with information to help you make the best possible food choices and take steps toward reducing your weight and increasing your health. Refer to it often.

Food Item	Serving Size	Calories	Fat	Protein	Carbs	Fiber	Cycle
A							
Alfalfa sprouts	1 cup	10	0	0	2	0	3–4
Almond milk	1 cup	60	2.5	1	8	1	3–4
Almonds, roasted	1 oz. (12 nuts)	169	15	6	6	6	3–4
Amaranth	½ cup	360	6	14	62	14	2–4
Apples, w/ skin	1 medium	72	0	0	19	3	1–4
Apricots	1 apricot	17	0	0	4	1	3–4
Artichoke	1 artichoke	76	0	5	17	9	1–4
Artichoke hearts	2 pieces	30	0	1	7	2	1–4
Arugula	1 cup	4	0	1	1	0	1–4
Asparagus	1 spear	2	0	0	1	0	1–4
Avocados	¼ fruit	136	12.5	2	7	6	3–4

302 *The 17 Day Diet Workbook*

Food Item	Serving Size	Calories	Fat	Protein	Carbs	Fiber	Cycle
B							
Bacon, Canadian	1 slice	43	2	6	0	0	2–4
Bamboo shoots	1 cup	41	1	4	8	3	3–4
Bananas	1 med., 7–8"	105	0	1	27	3	3–4
Barley, pearled, cooked	½ cup	97	0	2	22	3	2–4
Beans, adzuki, cooked	½ cup	147	0	8	14	4	2–4
Beans, black, cooked	½ cup	113	0	7	20	7	2–4
Beans, cranberry, cooked	½ cup	120	0	8	21	9	2–4
Beans, fava, canned	½ cup	91	0	7	15	5	2–4
Beans, French, cooked	1 cup	228	0	12	42	16	2–4
Beans, great northern, cooked	½ cup	105	0	7	18	6	2–4
Beans, kidney, cooked	½ cup	112	0	7	20	5	2–4
Beans, lima, canned	½ cup	95	0	6	18	5	2–4
Beans, lima, cooked	½ cup	108	0	7	20	7	2–4
Beans, navy, cooked	½ cup	127	0	7	24	10	2–4
Beans, pink, cooked	½ cup	126	0	7	24	4	2–4
Beans, pinto, cooked	½ cup	122	0	7	22	7	2–4
Beans, small white, cooked	½ cup	127	0	8	23	9	2–4
Beans, snap, green, cooked	1 cup	44	0	2	10	4	2–4
Beans, snap, yellow, cooked	1 cup	44	0	2	10	4	2–4
Beans, white, cooked	½ cup	125	0	8	23	5	2–4
Beans, yellow	½ cup	127	1	8	24	9	3–4
Beef, eye of the round	3 oz.	170	7	24	0	0	2–4
Beef, flank	3 oz.	180	9	23	0	0	2–4
Beef, ground, 95% lean, raw	3 oz.	145	6	22	0	0	2–4
Beef, sirloin	3 oz.	160	6	26	0	0	2–4

Food Item	Serving Size	Calories	Fat	Protein	Carbs	Fiber	Cycle
Beef, top loin	3 oz.	160	7	23	0	0	2–4
Beef, top round	3 oz.	158	5	27	0	0	2–4
Beets	1 beet	35	0	2	8	4	2–4
Bread, cracked wheat	1 slice	65	1	2	12	1	2–4
Bread, pita	2 oz.	150	1	3	30	0	2–4
Bread, pumpernickel	1 slice	75	1	3	15	2	2–4
Bread, rice bran	1 oz.	69	1	3	12	1	2–4
Bread, sandwich slice	1 slice	70	1	2	13	1	3–4
Breadfruit	1 cup	235	3	7	7	7	2–4
Broad beans, cooked	1 cup	187	1	13	33	9	2–4
Broccoli, cooked	1 cup	55	0	4	11	5	1–4
Broccoli sprouts	1 cup	31	0	3	6	2	3–4
Brussels sprouts, cooked	1 cup	56	1	4	11	4	1–4
Buckwheat groats, roasted, cooked	½ cup	77	0	3	17	3	2–4
Bulgur wheat, cooked	½ cup	160	0	5	34	4	2–4
C							
Cabbage, all varieties	1 cup, shredded	17	1	1	4	2	1–4
Canadian bacon	2 slices	89	4	12	0	0	3–4
Carrots	1 medium	65	0	1	15	4	1–4
Cashew nuts	1 oz.	157	12	5	9	1	3–4
Cauliflower, cooked	1 cup	29	0	3	5	3	1–4
Celery, raw, chopped	1 cup	14	0	3	1	2	1–4
Chard, Swiss	1 cup	7	0	1	1	1	1–4
Cheese, Brie	2 oz.	190	16	12	2	0	3–4
Cheese, Camembert	2 oz.	180	14	10	0	0	3–4
Cheese, cheddar, low fat	2 oz.	98	4	14	1	0	3–4
Cheese, cottage, 2%	½ cup	101	2	15	4	0	3–4
Cheese, edam	2 oz.	202	16	14	1	0	3–4
Cheese, feta, reduced fat	2 oz.	117	7	12	2	0	3–4

Food Item	Serving Size	Calories	Fat	Protein	Carbs	Fiber	Cycle
Cheese, fontina	2 oz.	221	18	15	1	0	3–4
Cheese, goat	2 oz.	256	20	17	1	0	3–4
Cheese, goat, semisoft	2 oz.	206	17	12	1	0	3–4
Cheese, mozzarella, part skim	2 oz.	144	9	14	2	0	3–4
Cheese, Parmesan, grated	2 tbsp.	43	3	4	0	0	3–4
Cheese, Parmigiano-reggiano, grated	2 tbsp.	40	3	4	0	0	3–4
Cheese, ricotta, light	½ cup	120	5	10	6	0	3–4
Cheese, Roquefort, reduced fat	2 oz.	49	2	1	8	0	3–4
Cheese, string, light	1 string	50	3	6	1	0	3–4
Cheese, Swiss, reduced fat	2 oz.	101	3	16	2	0	3–4
Cherries, sour	8 pieces	30	0	1	7	2	3–4
Cherries, sweet	8 pieces	30	0	2	7	2	3–4
Chicken breast, w/o skin	½ breast	130	2	27	0	0	1–4
Chicken, Cornish game hen, meat only	1 bird	295	9	51	0	0	2–4
Chicken, dark meat, w/o skin	1 cup, diced	287	14	38	0	0	4
Chicken, light meat, w/o skin	1 cup, diced	214	6	38	0	0	1–4
Chickpeas, cooked	1 cup	269	4	15	45	13	2–4
Chicory greens	1 cup, chopped	41	1	3	9	7	1–4
Clams, steamed or boiled	1 cup	138	2	24	5	0	2–4
Cold cereals, All-Bran	1 cup	160	2	8	46	20	3–4
Cold cereals, All-Bran Bran Buds	1 cup	140	2	4	48	26	3–4
Cold cereals, Fiber One	1 cup	120	2	4	50	28	3–4
Cold cereals, gluten-free	¾ cup	200	3	7	42	6	3–4

Food Item	Serving Size	Calories	Fat	Protein	Carbs	Fiber	Cycle
Collards	1 cup, chopped	11	0	1	2	1	1–4
Conch, baked or broiled	1 cup, sliced	165	2	33	2	0	2–4
Corn, sweet, white	1 ear	77	1	3	17	2	2–4
Corn, sweet, yellow	1 ear	77	1	3	17	2	2–4
Couscous, cooked	1 cup	176	0	6	37	0	2–4
Cowpeas (black-eyed peas), cooked	1 cup	160	1	5	34	8	2–4
Crab, Alaskan king, raw	1 leg	144	1	32	0	0	2–4
Crab, blue, canned	1 cup	134	2	28	0	0	2–4
Crab, Dungeness, cooked	1 crab	140	2	28	1	0	2–4
Crackers, melba toast	1 cup	129	1	4	25	2	4
Crackers, rye	1 cracker	37	0	1	9	3	4
Crackers, wheat	1 cracker	60	9	0	0	1	4
Crackers, whole wheat	1 cracker	18	1	0	3	0	4
Cranberries	1 cup, whole	44	0	0	12	4	1–4
Crayfish, wild	8 crayfish	21	0	4	0	0	2–4
Cream of Wheat	¾ cup	98	0	3	21	1	2–4
Cucumber	1 cucumber	45	0	2	11	2	1–4
Cucumber, peeled	1 cup, sliced	14	0	1	3	1	3–4
Currants, black	1 cup	71	1	2	17	0	3–4
Currants, red & white	1 cup	63	0	2	16	5	1–4
D							
Dandelion greens	1 cup, chopped	25	0	2	5	2	1–4
E							
Egg, hard-boiled	1 cup, chopped	211	14	17	2	0	1–4
Egg noodles, cooked	½ cup	107	1	4	20	1	3–4
Egg, poached	1 large	74	5	6	0	0	1–4
Egg, scrambled	1 cup	365	27	24	5	0	1–4
Egg substitute, liquid	1 tbsp.	13	1	2	0	0	1–4
Egg white, raw	1 large	17	0	4	0	0	1–4

Food Item	Serving Size	Calories	Fat	Protein	Carbs	Fiber	Cycle
Eggplant	1 eggplant	110	10	5	26	16	1–4
Elderberries	1 cup	106	1	1	27	10	1–4
Endive	1 head	87	1	6	17	16	1–4
F							
Farina, cooked	½ cup	235	0	1.5	12	0	2–4
Fennel	1 cup, sliced	27	0	1	6	3	3–4
Figs	1 medium	37	0	0	10	2	3–4
Figs, dried	1 fig	21	0	0	5	1	3–4
Fish, bluefin tuna	3 oz.	122	4	20	0	0	1–4
Fish, bluefish	3 oz.	105	4	17	0	0	1–4
Fish, butterfish	3 oz.	124	7	15	0	0	1–4
Fish, carp	3 oz.	108	5	15	0	0	1–4
Fish, catfish	3 oz.	81	2	14	0	0	1–4
Fish, cod, Atlantic	3 oz.	70	1	15	0	0	1–4
Fish, croaker, Atlantic	3 oz.	88	3	15	0	0	1–4
Fish, flounder	3 oz.	77	1	16	0	0	1–4
Fish, haddock	3 oz.	74	1	16	0	0	1–4
Fish, halibut	3 oz.	94	2	18	0	0	1–4
Fish, herring, Atlantic	3 oz.	134	8	15	0	0	1–4
Fish, herring, Pacific	3 oz.	166	12	14	0	0	1–4
Fish, mackerel, Atlantic	3 oz.	174	12	16	0	0	1–4
Fish, mackerel, king	3 oz.	89	2	17	0	0	1–4
Fish, mackerel, Pacific	3 oz.	134	7	17	0	0	1–4
Fish, mackerel, Spanish	3 oz.	118	5	16	0	0	1–4
Fish, milkfish	3 oz.	126	6	18	0	0	1–4
Fish, monkfish	3 oz.	65	1	12	0	0	1–4
Fish, ocean perch, Atlantic	3 oz.	80	1	16	0	0	1–4
Fish, perch, mixed species	3 oz.	77	1	17	0	0	1–4
Fish, pike, northern	3 oz.	75	1	16	0	0	1–4
Fish, pollock, Atlantic	3 oz.	78	1	17	0	0	1–4
Fish, rainbow smelt	3 oz.	82	2	15	0	0	1–4

Food Item	Serving Size	Calories	Fat	Protein	Carbs	Fiber	Cycle
Fish, rockfish, Pacific	3 oz.	80	1	16	0	0	1–4
Fish, roe, mixed species	1 tbsp.	20	10	3	0	0	1–4
Fish, sablefish	3 oz.	166	13	11	0	0	1–4
Fish, salmon, Atlantic, farmed	3 oz.	156	9	17	0	0	1–4
Fish, salmon, Atlantic, wild	3 oz.	121	5	17	0	0	1–4
Fish, salmon, Chinook	3 oz.	152	9	17	0	0	1–4
Fish, salmon, pink	3 oz.	99	3	17	0	0	1–4
Fish, sea bass, mixed species	3 oz.	82	2	16	0	0	1–4
Fish, sea trout, mixed species	3 oz.	88	3	14	0	0	1–4
Fish, shad	3 oz.	167	12	14	0	0	1–4
Fish, skipjack tuna	3 oz.	88	1	19	0	0	1–4
Fish, snapper, mixed species	3 oz.	85	1	17	0	0	1–4
Fish, striped bass	3 oz.	82	2	15	0	0	1–4
Fish, striped mullet	3 oz.	99	3	16	0	0	1–4
Fish, sturgeon, mixed species	3 oz.	89	3	14	0	0	1–4
Fish, tilapia	3 oz.	108	2	22	0	0	1–4
Fish, trout	3 oz.	126	6	18	0	0	1–4
Fish, white sucker	3 oz.	78	2	14	0	0	1–4
Fish, whitefish	3 oz.	114	5	16	0	0	1–4
Fish, wolffish, Atlantic	3 oz.	82	2	15	0	0	1–4
Fish, yellowfin tuna	3 oz.	93	1	20	0	0	1–4
Flaxseed oil	1 tbsp.	120	14	0	0	0	1–4
G							
Garden cress, raw	1 cup	16	0	1	3	1	1–4
Garlic	1 clove	4	0	0	1	0	1–4
Granola, low fat	½ cup	190	2.5	4	40	3	3–4
Grape leaves	4 leaves	11	0	1	2	0	3–4
Grapefruit	½ fruit	50	0	1	12	3	1–4
Grapes, red	1 cup	106	0	1	28	1	1–4
Grits	¾ cup	107	0	3	24	1	2–4
Guavas	1 fruit	37	1	1	8	3	3–4

Food Item	Serving Size	Calories	Fat	Protein	Carbs	Fiber	Cycle
H							
Hazelnuts, dry roasted	1 oz.	183	18	4	5	3	3–4
Hominy, canned, white	1 cup	119	2	2	24	4	2–4
Hominy, canned, yellow	1 cup	115	1	2	23	4	2–4
J							
Japanese soba noodles, cooked	1 cup	113	0	6	24	2	3–4
Jicama, sliced	1 cup	46	0	1	11	6	3–4
K							
Kale	1 cup, chopped	34	1	2	7	1	1–4
Kefir, low fat, plain	1 cup	120	2	14	12	3	1–4
Kiwi	1 medium	45	0	2	11	5	3–4
Kohlrabi, cooked	1 cup	29	0	2	7	1	3–4
Kumquats	1 fruit	13	0	0	3	1	3–4
L							
Lamb, leg, shank half	3 oz.	156	9	15	0	0	2–4
Lamb, leg, sirloin half	3 oz.	222	18	15	0	0	2–4
Lamb, loin, choice, raw	3 oz.	237	18	15	0	0	2–4
Leeks	1 leek	54	0	1	13	2	1–4
Lemons w/ peel	1 fruit	22	0	1	12	5	1–4
Lentils, cooked	1 cup	230	1	18	40	16	2–4
Lettuce, green leaf	1 cup, shredded	5	0	1	1	1	1–4
Lettuce, iceberg	1 cup, shredded	10	0	1	2	1	1–4
Lettuce, red leaf	1 cup, shredded	3	0	0	0	0	1–4
Lettuce, romaine	1 cup, shredded	8	0	1	2	1	1–4
Limes	1 fruit	20	0	1	7	2	1–4
Lobster, northern, raw	1 lobster	135	1	28	1	0	2–4
M							
Macadamia nuts	1 oz. (10–12 nuts)	203	22	2	4	2	3–4

Food Item	Serving Size	Calories	Fat	Protein	Carbs	Fiber	Cycle
Mangos	1 fruit	135	1	1	35	4	3–4
Margarine, fat-free spread	1 tbsp.	6	0	0	1	0	3–4
Mayonnaise	1 tbsp.	100	11	0	0	0	3–4
Mayonnaise, light	1 tbsp.	50	5	0	0	0	3–4
Milk, buttermilk, cultured, reduced fat	1 cup	137	5	10	13	0	3–4
Milk, dry, nonfat, instant	⅓ cup dry	82	0	8	12	0	3–4
Milk, 1% low fat	1 cup	102	2	8	12	0	3–4
Milk, 2% low fat	1 cup	138	5	10	14	0	3–4
Millet	1 cup	207	1.7	6	41	3	2–4
Miso soup, reduced sodium	½ cup	273	8	16	36	7	1–4
Mushrooms	1 cup, pieces	15	0	2	2	1	1–4
Mushrooms, enoki	1 large	2	2	0	0	0	1–4
Mushrooms, oyster	1 large	55	1	6	9	4	1–4
Mushrooms, portobello	1 large	22	0	2	4	2	1–4
Mushrooms, shiitake	1 mushroom	11	0	0	3	0	1–4
Mussels, blue, raw	1 cup	129	3	18	6	0	2–4
Mustard greens	1 cup, chopped	15	0	2	3	2	1–4
Mustard, prepared, yellow	1 tsp.	3	0	0	0	0	1–4
N							
Nectarines	1 fruit	60	0	1	14	2	1–4
Nopales, cubed, cooked	1 cup	35	0	1	9	3	3–4
O							
Oat bran	½ cup	118	3	8	31	7	2–4
Oatmeal, instant, prepared w/ water	½ cup	65	1	3	11	2	2–4
Oil, canola	1 tbsp.	124	14	0	0	0	3–4
Oil, olive	1 tbsp.	119	14	0	0	0	1–4
Oil, sesame	1 tbsp.	120	14	0	0	0	3–4
Oil, vegetable, walnut	1 tbsp.	120	14	0	0	0	3–4
Okra	1 cup	31	0	2	7	3	1–4
Onions	1 cup, chopped	67	0	2	16	2	1–4
Onions, sweet	1 onion	106	0	3	25	3	1–4

Food Item	Serving Size	Calories	Fat	Protein	Carbs	Fiber	Cycle
Oranges	1 large	86	0	2	22	4	1–4
Oyster, eastern, raw	3 oz.	50	1	4	5	0	2–4
Oyster, Pacific, raw	3 oz.	69	2	8	4	0	2–4
P							
Papayas	1 cup, cubed	55	0	1	14	3	3–4
Parsley	1 cup	22	1	2	4	2	1–4
Parsley, dried	1 tsp.	1	0	0	0	0	1–4
Parsnips	1 cup, sliced	100	0	2	24	7	2–4
Pasta, corn, cooked	1 cup	176	1	4	39	7	3–4
Pasta, plain, cooked	1 cup	197	1	7	40	2	3–4
Pasta, spinach, cooked	1 cup	195	1	8	38	2	3–4
Peaches	1 large	61	0	1	15	2	1–4
Peapods	1 cup	83	1	6	14	5	3–4
Peanuts, dry roasted w/ salt	1 oz.	166	14	7	6	2	3–4
Pears	1 pear	121	0	1	32	7	1–4
Pears, Asian	1 pear	116	1	1	29	10	1–4
Peas, green, fresh, cooked	1 cup	134	0	9	25	9	2–4
Peas, green, frozen, cooked	1 cup	125	0	8	23	9	2–4
Peas, split, cooked	1 cup	231	1	16	41	16	2–4
Pecans	1 oz. (20 halves)	196	20	3	40	3	3–4
Peppers, chili, green	1 cup	29	0	1	6	2	3–4
Peppers, chili, red	1 pepper	18	0	1	4	1	3–4
Peppers, jalapeño	1 pepper	4	0	0	1	0	3–4
Peppers, sweet, green	1 medium	24	0	1	6	2	1–4
Peppers, sweet, red	1 medium	31	0	1	7	2	1–4
Peppers, sweet, yellow	1 medium	32	0	1	8	1	1–4
Pheasant, breast, w/o skin	3 oz.	113	3	21	0	0	3–4
Pineapple	1 fruit	227	1	3	60	7	3–4
Pistachio nuts	1 oz. (49 kernels)	161	13	6	8	3	3–4

Food Item	Serving Size	Calories	Fat	Protein	Carbs	Fiber	Cycle
Pita bread, whole wheat	1 pita	170	2	6	35	5	3–4
Plantains	1 medium	218	1	2	57	4	3–4
Plums	1 fruit	30	0	1	8	1	1–4
Polenta	½ cup	220	2	2	24	1	2–4
Pomegranates	1 fruit	105	1	2	26	1	3–4
Popcorn, air-popped	1 cup	31	0	1	6	1	3–4
Pork, loin, center loin, cooked	3 oz.	199	11	22	0	0	2–4
Pork, loin, sirloin, cooked	3 oz.	176	8	24	0	0	2–4
Pork, loin, tenderloin, cooked	3 oz.	147	5	24	0	0	2–4
Pork, loin, top loin, cooked	3 oz.	192	10	24	0	0	2–4
Pork, loin, whole, cooked	3 oz.	211	12	23	0	0	2–4
Potatoes	1 medium	164	0	4	37	5	2–4
Potatoes, baked, w/ skin	1 medium	160	0	4	37	4	2–4
Potatoes, baked, w/o skin	1 medium	143	0	3	35	3	2–4
Potatoes, red	1 medium	153	0	4	34	4	2–4
Potatoes, russet	1 medium	168	0	5	39	3	2–4
Potatoes, white	1 medium	149	0	4	34	5	2–4
Prunes, unsweetened	4 prunes	100	0	1	24	3	1–4
Pumpkin	1 cup	30	0	1	8	1	2–4
Pumpkin, canned	1 cup	83	1	3	20	7	2–4
Q							
Quail, breast, w/o skin	3 oz.	105	3	19	0	0	3–4
Quinoa, cooked	½ cup	127	2	5	24	2	2–4
R							
Radicchio	1 cup, shredded	9	0	1	2	0	1–4
Radishes	1 cup, sliced	19	0	1	4	2	3–4
Raspberries	1 cup	64	1	2	15	8	1–4
Rhubarb	1 cup, diced	26	0	1	6	2	3–4
Rice, basmati	½ cup	140	2	3	31	2	2–4
Rice, brown	½ cup	127	1	3	27	2	2–4
Rice milk	1 cup	120	3	1	23	0	3–4

Food Item	Serving Size	Calories	Fat	Protein	Carbs	Fiber	Cycle
Rice, wild	½ cup	83	0	3	17	2	2–4
Rutabaga	1 cup, cubed	50	0	2	11	4	3–4
S							
Salad dressing, bacon and tomato	1 tbsp.	49	5	0	0	0	3–4
Salad dressing, blue cheese	1 tbsp.	77	8	1	1	0	3–4
Salad dressing, Caesar	1 tbsp.	78	9	0	1	0	3–4
Salad dressing, coleslaw	1 tbsp.	61	5	0	4	0	3–4
Salad dressing, French	1 tbsp.	71	7	9	2	0	3–4
Salad dressing, honey Dijon	1 tbsp.	58	5	1	3	1	3–4
Salad dressing, Italian	1 tbsp.	43	4	0	2	0	3–4
Salad dressing, light varieties	2 tbsp.	23	2	0	1	0	3–4
Salad dressing, mayonnaise	1 tbsp.	57	5	0	3.5	0	3–4
Salad dressing, peppercorn	1 tbsp.	76	8	0	1	0	3–4
Salad dressing, ranch	1 tbsp.	25	8	0	0	0	3–4
Salad dressing, Russian	1 tbsp.	76	8	0	2	0	3–4
Salad dressing, Thousand Island	1 tbsp.	58	6	0	2	0	3–4
Salsa, w/o oil	2 tbsp.	15	0	0	4	0	1–4
Sauce, marinara	1 cup	185	6	5	28	1	1–4
Sauce, salsa	1 cup	70	0	4	16	4	1–4
Sauce, soy	1 tbsp.	10	0	0	0	0	1–4
Sauce, steak	1 tbsp.	25	0	0	6	0	1–4
Sauce, teriyaki	1 tbsp.	15	0	17	2	0	1–4
Sauce, Worcestershire	1 cup	184	0	0	54	0	1–4
Sauerkraut	½ cup	25	0	1	5	4	3–4
Sausage, turkey	1 link, 1 oz.	67	5	4	0.5	0	3–4
Scallions, chopped	½ cup	18	0	1	4	2	1–4
Scallops	1 scallop	26	0	5	1	0	2–4
Shallots	1 tbsp., chopped	7	0	0	2	0	1–4

Food Item	Serving Size	Calories	Fat	Protein	Carbs	Fiber	Cycle
Shrimp, mixed species, raw	1 medium shrimp	6	0	1	0	0	2–4
Soy burger	1 patty	125	4	13	9	3	1–4
Soy milk	1 cup	127	5	11	12	3	3–4
Soybeans, green, cooked	1 cup	254	12	22	12	7	2–4
Soybeans, nuts, roasted, dry	¼ cup	194	9	17	14	3	3–4
Spaghetti, spinach, cooked	1 cup	182	1	6	37	2	1–4
Spaghetti, whole wheat, cooked	1 cup	174	1	7	37	6	1–4
Spinach	1 cup	7	0	1	1	1	1–4
Squash, summer	1 cup, sliced	18	0	1	4	1	3–4
Squash, winter	1 cup, cubed	39	0	1	10	2	2–4
Squid, mixed species, raw	1 oz.	26	0	4	1	0	2–4
Stock, beef	1 cup	31	0	5	3	0	1–4
Stock, chicken	1 cup	86	3	6	9	0	1–4
Strawberries	1 cup	49	1	1	12	3	1–4
Sunflower seeds	1 tbsp.	47	4	2	2	1	3–4
Sweet potato	1 cup, cubed	114	0	2	27	4	2–4
T							
Tangelo	1 medium	47	0	1	12	2	3–4
Tangerine	1 large	52	3	2	6	0	3–4
Taro, cooked	½ cup	94	0	0	23	3.4	2–4
Tofu, firm	½ cup	183	11	20	5	3	1–4
Tofu, soft	½ cup	76	5	8	2	0	1–4
Tomato paste, canned	½ cup	107	1	6	25	6	1–4
Tomato sauce, canned	1 cup	78	1	3	18	4	1–4
Tomatoes, canned, crushed	1 cup	82	1	4	19	5	1–4
Tomatoes, green	1 cup, chopped	41	0	2	9	2	1–4
Tomatoes, orange	1 cup, chopped	25	0	2	5	1	1–4
Tomatoes, red	1 cup, chopped	32	0	2	7	2	1–4
Tortilla, whole wheat, 10"	1 tortilla	120	5	2	16	1	3–4
Turkey bacon	2 slices	70	5	4	0	0	3–4

Food Item	Serving Size	Calories	Fat	Protein	Carbs	Fiber	Cycle
Turkey, breast, skinless, meat only, roasted	4 oz.	153	1	34	0	0	1–4
Turkey, dark meat, skinless, meat only, roasted	4 oz.	183	5	33	0	0	4
Turkey, deli sliced, white meat	1 oz.	30	1	5	1	0	1–4
Turnip greens, chopped	1 cup	18	0	1	4	2	1–4
Turnips, cubed	1 cup	36	0	1	8	2	2–4
V							
Veal cutlet	3 oz.	128	3	24	0	0	2–4
W							
Walnuts	1 oz. (14 halves)	185	19	4	4	2	3–4
Watercress	1 cup, chopped	4	0	1	0	0	1–4
Watermelon	1 cup, diced	46	0	1	12	1	3–4
Wine, red	3.5-oz. glass	74	0	0	2	0	3–4
Wine, white	3.5-oz. glass	70	0	0	1	0	3–4
Y							
Yakult	1 bottle	50	0	0	0	0	1–4
Yam	1 cup, cubed	177	0	2	42	6	2–4
Yogurt, fruit, low fat	8-oz. container	118	0	6	24	0	1–4
Yogurt, fruit, whole milk	8-oz. container	250	6	9	38	0	1–4
Yogurt, plain, low fat	8-oz. container	110	4	8	7	0	1–4
Yogurt, plain, whole milk	8-oz. container	138	7	12	11	0	1–4
Z							
Zucchini	1 medium	46	0	2	10	1	3–4